A MOTHER KNOWS

JOEY DLAMINI

A
MOTHER
KNOWS

Finding Courage and Confidence to Take Ownership of
Your Child's Developmental Journey

INSPIRED
PUBLISHING

A Mother Knows
Finding Courage and Confidence to Take Ownership of Your
Child's Developmental Journey
First Edition, First Impression 2025
ISBN: 978-0-6398535-0-5
Copyright © Joey Dlamini

Published by:
Inspired Publishing
PO Box 82058 | Southdale | 2135, Johannesburg, South Africa
Email: info@inspiredpublishing.co.za
www.inspiredpublishing.co.za

Edited by: Eloise Scoble

Dedication

As we conclude this chapter of our ongoing journey, I would like to dedicate this writing to my daughter, whose resilience, strength, and tenacity continue to inspire me every day. Your ability to rise above challenges and embrace life with courage is a testament to your incredible spirit. You remind me that even in the face of adversity, there is always a reason to hope and strive for a better tomorrow.

As I reflect on the strides I have taken amidst the pain, frustration, and uncertainty, I commend myself for my unwavering determination and commitment to your well-being. Each step forward has been a testament to my love for you and a reminder that growth often comes through struggle.

I extend my heartfelt gratitude to my husband, whose unwavering support and partnership have made this journey lighter and more meaningful. I also want to acknowledge our extended family, whose love and encouragement have been invaluable. To your brothers, who have stood by your side throughout this journey, and to all our family members who have assisted and continue to support us, your kindness and compassion have not gone unnoticed. As we look ahead, I am filled with hope and excitement for your future. It shines brightly, filled with endless possibilities and opportunities. Together, we will continue to navigate this journey, celebrating every victory, big and small, and fostering a life rich with love, joy, and fulfillment.

Contents

Dedication 5

Acknowledgments 7

Foreword..9

How It All Started 11

My Worst Fears Confirmed.......................................22

You Are Allowed To Change Your Mind....................28

Toxic Positivity 32

Living While Waiting For Life-Changing Surgery.......38

New Year, New Hope 43

Life Post-Surgery 52

Reflections Four Months Post-Surgery 65

A New Chapter: Big School.......................................75

Navigating Nerves And Expectations 84

A Painful Mother's Day...96

Maybe I'm Having A Pity Party................................106

What If The Lord Revealed The Hidden Parts Of Your Child So That They Would Receive The Help That They Needed? 117

Conversation With Speech Therapist Nazmeerah......124

For The One Who No Longer Trusts Her Intuition.................132

The Journey Continues...154

Recap – The Experts..157

Acknowledgments

First and foremost, I want to thank my Heavenly Father, who has been my constant source of strength throughout this journey. I know that without His guidance and the enabling power of the Holy Spirit, I could not have accomplished this. Every step has been a testament to His grace, and for that, I am eternally grateful.

To my beloved husband, my Mumuzela, look at how deeply God has loved us by giving you to us as the head of this family. Your steadfastness and unwavering love have been a fortress for us. Thank you for all the giants you face daily for our sake, for your quiet strength, and for leading our family with wisdom, courage, and faith. I could not have asked for a better partner on this journey.

To my wonderful children, my squad: Reokesitswe, Tshiamo, and Asante, thank you for bringing so much joy and meaning to this parenting journey. You have made it easier in ways you may never fully understand.
Reokesitswe and Tshiamo, to you especially, thank you for your boundless love and support for your sister, for standing by her, and for reminding me daily of the beauty of sibling love and unity.

Each of you brings light into our lives, and I am so proud to be your mother.

Finally, to everyone who has shared their stories with me, who has lifted me up in prayer, and who has offered words of encouragement along the way—thank you. Your kindness, wisdom, and faith have sustained me in moments when I needed them most. I am because you are; your support has been a pillar that helped me persevere.

From the depths of my heart, thank you.

Foreword

Imagine being a mother who has faced the unimaginable: the loss of a child, the diagnosis of a disability, and the uncertainty of what the future holds. Yet, in the midst of chaos and uncertainty, you discover a profound truth: a mother knows.

As I reflect on my own journey as a mother, I am reminded of the twists and turns that have shaped me into the person I am today. From the pain of pregnancy loss to the joy of raising two beautiful children—one with special needs and one developing typically—I've learned that motherhood is a journey that defies expectations and redefines love.

That is why I am so passionate about this book, *A Mother Knows*. It is a powerful reminder that motherhood is not a one-size-fits-all journey. It celebrates the diversity, complexity, and beauty of motherly love. Through its pages, I have found solace, inspiration, and a deeper understanding of my own experiences as a mother.

As we embark on this journey together, I invite you to join me in exploring the complexities, nuances, and beauty of motherhood.

Within the pages of this book, may you find inspiration, comfort, and a deeper appreciation of the transformative power of motherly love. Let us walk this path together, and may our shared experiences and insights illuminate the journey.

— Sibongile Alice Masemola: A Mother, Wife, Sister, and Friend.
I am a storyteller, an advocate for neurodiverse children and individuals, and a passionate voice for inclusion and acceptance.

1

How It All Started

Motherhood is a journey that often defies logic, shaped by an unspoken bond and a powerful intuition. From the moment a child is born, a mother is also born—a transformation as profound as the birth itself. It's not only the beginning of a new life for the child but the beginning of an entirely new identity for the woman. She steps into a role filled with immense love, responsibility, and a sense of connection that goes beyond the physical. This bond creates an emotional and spiritual link between mother and child, a link that only deepens as the days go by.

While those who are not mothers—or are not mothers yet—may dismiss or question the validity of a mother's intuition, attempting to undermine this deeply personal journey, there is a truth that remains unchanged: a mother's knowing is unlike any other. The moment her child enters the world, a mother is instinctively equipped with a profound sense of awareness, an inexplicable inner compass that guides her. It's a sense that cannot be taught or learned, only felt—an awakening to a new dimension of life.

There is a unique wisdom that only a mother carries—an innate understanding that transcends words, time, and experience. A mother's knowledge is not something learned in books or by instruction; it is felt, deeply woven into the very fabric of her being. She anticipates her child's needs even before they are expressed, offering silent strength in moments of uncertainty and providing unwavering care and protection without ever seeking anything in return. As a baby learns and grows, so too does the mother, evolving with her child, trusting her instincts to navigate the unknown.

Even though society has worked so hard to make mothers doubt their intuition, instinct, and gut feelings, often making them feel as though they are overreacting—gaslighting them into questioning their own judgment—there is one thing I have observed and continue to experience: a mama has a deep, unshakeable knowing of what is happening with her children. This understanding sometimes transcends what can be explained by human reason; it is a knowing that runs deep, beyond what others may comprehend.

Society often influences women to doubt their intuition in several ways, and while these influences may be subtle to some, they can be glaring to others. Frequently, it is not that someone has explicitly stated that your instincts are off-key; rather, it is the culture and background from which you come that have laid this foundation in a woman long before she even has children. Many cultures propagate the notion that emotions are irrational or that women are overly emotional. This pervasive narrative can lead women to question their feelings and instincts, viewing them as unreliable or unfounded. Historically, women's roles have been confined to the domestic sphere, and while this fact should strengthen their belief in their own intuition and its validity, any instinctual knowledge associated with that role has been trivialised. The perception of "just" being a mother implies that expressing gut feelings is somehow irrational, rendering women's insights less valid than those of men.

Yet, when a man claims that he can "feel" that the "drive in his car is different" and suspects something may be wrong, he is typically given the benefit of the doubt to have the issue checked by a mechanic. The mechanic will generally verify whether the vehicle needs attention because, ultimately, allowing "the problem" to linger can lead to a very expensive repair down the line. Conversely, when a mother expresses the same instinct regarding her child, **society encourages her to wait and see if the child will simply "grow out of it,"** as though she has no concern for the potential damage that may occur if left unchecked for too long.

Another factor that contributes to women doubting their intuition is traditional education, which has often emphasised analytical thinking over emotional intelligence. This emphasis leads women to prioritise logical reasoning at the expense of intuitive understanding, thereby diminishing the value placed on feelings and instincts.

Additionally, many women overlook the impact of social comparison. The rise of social media has intensified the pressure on women to compare themselves with others. Observing curated portrayals of parenting or personal achievements can sow seeds of self-doubt, making women feel inadequate and prompting them to question their own choices and instincts. This culture of comparison creates a sense that admitting we sense a problem with our children makes us bad parents. If our children do not follow the route deemed "successful" in conventional child-rearing, we may internalise a feeling of failure, particularly as mothers.

Despite the many ways society influences women to doubt their intuition, there are moments in life that reaffirm our innate sense of knowing. For me, this happened on the day I discovered I was pregnant with my daughter. I vividly remember waking up with an overwhelming certainty. One of my very first thoughts that morning was, *I am pregnant.* No, I wasn't experiencing morning sickness, and I hadn't even missed my period. Yet, when I woke up that morning, I just knew. Later that evening, I took the pregnancy test, and it confirmed what I had already instinctively known. That moment only solidified my belief in the incredible intuition that mothers possess—a knowing that begins the moment a baby is conceived and only grows stronger from the day of birth.

Why am I sharing this story? Because I want you to know and always remember that this is only one of the very few things that comes without prior experience. This intuition is innate, waiting to be embraced and nurtured. While it is true that intuition needs to be practised and you must learn to trust yourself, it does not require you to have been a mother for a significant period or to have had two or three children. You need no qualifications to trust your gut as a mother.

I hadn't even held my baby in my arms when I first experienced this deep sense of knowing. It didn't begin once I *knew for sure* I was pregnant. This intuition came as a result of conceiving itself. It seemed as though it came in tandem with conception, a natural awareness that emerged from the very moment life began inside me. I am telling you this because I am hoping that it will remind you **of the instances where you knew something, but you took it for granted or you thought that it was a normal human reaction.**

Before I had my daughter, I was convinced that I was doing just fine. I was actively pursuing my goals, and I truly believed that I was living as my most authentic self. I thought I had everything figured out. However, watching her grow has unearthed parts of me that I had long forgotten or perhaps deliberately tried to hide. It's as though her presence brought out truths within me that I hadn't even realised were buried. Her growth became a mirror, reflecting not only her own journey but also the layers of myself that were waiting to be rediscovered.

I realised that on my journey of becoming, I had lost my confidence in myself. I no longer trusted my inner voice and sought confirmation from others to believe that what I was doing was right or to validate my inner intuition. I have never been one to obsess over whether my kids reached their milestones on time; reflecting on it now, I recognise the privilege I had with my first children. They simply grew up without the struggle that often accompanies learning and development. I don't recall teaching them to write their names, recite the alphabet, count, or even speak; I would merely notice their progress and reinforce those lessons when necessary. Essentially, they either learned on their own or from teachers and other significant figures in their lives. I assumed the same would hold true for their sister.

For the first two years, it seemed that her journey would mirror that of her brothers. She accomplished all her developmental tasks—as best as she could. However, as she approached her third birthday, I began to have concerns about her speech. While she was talking, her articulation of certain words was not clear. Do you know what I did? I waited for someone to tell me that I was overreacting—and they did. So, I temporarily stopped worrying and continued with my life as best as I could.

My daughter, determined to communicate, demonstrated remarkable creativity in her attempts to express herself. She often resorted to non-verbal communication to convey her messages. If we didn't understand her words, she would physically take us to the object she was referring to. I celebrated her ingenuity, even as that small voice inside me urged me to seek help. I remember discussing my concerns with my husband, and I could see the fear in his eyes. Together, we decided to hold on to hope that it was a passing stage. After all, kids are not all the same.

It wasn't that she wasn't talking at all; some of her words were just unclear, while others would surprise us with their fluency. We are a multilingual family—I'm Mopedi, my husband is Zulu, and the boys primarily speak English because of school. We noticed that my daughter was mixing languages in her sentences, often saying, "I want nyama" (meaning "I want meat"). Honestly, we were not worried; it was cute, and we laughed, believing that she would outgrow it, just as her brothers had.

When she went for her three-year immunisation, I thought the doctors would pick up on something, but they assured us she was fine. I am not blaming anyone; I am simply sharing how, despite having my own concerns, I still wanted someone in authority to tell me whether I was right or wrong. I was willing to trust someone who had observed my daughter for only a few minutes over my own instincts as her primary caregiver. After all, I am not an expert or a professional in child development, despite raising two kids and being surrounded by children throughout my entire 40 years of life. **I had lost trust in my heart knowledge because society often questioned it and deemed it insufficient.**
I often turned to Google for answers about my daughter's speech, but sometimes what I found didn't make sense to me. Other times, I felt like I was diagnosing her myself. I would watch how she played and did things and tried to figure out if she might have autism, but I could never be sure. I decided that if her speech wasn't more fluent by the time she turned four, I would take her to a professional.

Before her fourth birthday, I took her to the general practitioner because she had the flu. While we were there, I asked him for a referral because I was worried about her speech. He laughed it off and reassured me that I was overreacting after speaking with her for just a few seconds. She answered his questions, which made it seem like everything was fine. I left feeling unsure, thinking maybe I was overreacting if the doctor believed so. The truth is, I wasn't ready to hear any news other than that she was okay.

As a family, we continued on, and while she grew, she really tried her best but still struggled with some words. After she turned four years old, I started having conversations with different people to see if they noticed what I was noticing or heard what I was hearing. The fact that I felt the need for so many opinions showed that somewhere along my journey into adulthood, I had lost trust in myself. Maybe you're going through something similar.

This wasn't always the case; I remember being a very talkative child who asked a lot of questions. I questioned things that I did not understand. Some adults nurtured my curiosity and found it interesting, while others thought it was annoying. Those who didn't like it made sure that I knew their displeasure through the names they called me; names like "mosadinyana," which means "little woman." This was not a compliment; it was a way to dismiss me and shame my curiosity. Now, I wonder if those comments contributed to my uncertainty about my instincts.

It is with this in mind that I caution you, as an adult, to consider the words you use when speaking to children. Let's not be the reason they start doubting their intuition.

During that time, my daughter was attending a different crèche than the one she started with in the township. I truly believed that if there was anything wrong, they would let me know. Once again, I was seeking someone else's opinion to confirm or dismiss what my gut was telling me. I had always thought there was no need for her to start at a multiracial daycare because I wanted her to learn her mother tongue before being introduced to English. It also didn't make financial sense to pay so much for a daycare when they were still too young to actively learn.

An online friend opened my eyes to the fact that she had taken her children to a multiracial daycare not primarily for them to speak English, but for access to resources. She explained that these daycares often had speech therapists and occupational therapists who could identify issues early on, unlike many township daycares, which are mostly under-resourced. When she said this, I had an "aha" moment and felt a pang of regret that my well-intentioned but misguided reasoning might have put my daughter at a disadvantage. Instead of dwelling on my mistakes, I chose to forgive myself for not knowing better. If you find yourself in a similar situation, I encourage you to extend yourself some grace as well.

I decided to follow the same approach I used with her brothers. Rather than enrolling her in daycare when she was just one year old, I waited until she turned two. I believed daycare was more suitable for toddlers, a misconception I'm sure I'm not alone in having. Before that, she had stayed with her late great-grandmother, who loved being with her until I felt she needed to interact with other kids. This was during the COVID-19 pandemic in 2020 to 2021.

Like most children, when she started daycare, she often came home with a runny nose or a cough. Visiting the doctor became a regular occurrence for us. We assumed her immune system was just

19

adjusting to being around other kids. She would be home for a few days, recover, and then return to school, only to get sick again. We tried every multivitamin available, but she still caught colds. Eventually, we decided her immune system needed to learn how to fight off these illnesses. By the end of 2021, we decided to take her out of daycare because I felt the environment was too cold. However, the principal insisted that all the other kids were fine, making it seem like my daughter was the only one with a problem instead of working on a solution.

In February 2022, we enrolled her in a new daycare, with a huge playground and separate classes. It seemed promising, and I hoped she would thrive there. The daycare was absolutely beautiful, with small wooden tables and chairs and a large outdoor play area. I had high expectations.

At the end of the first term, I asked for her report, but I was informed that they only provide detailed reports twice a year. I noted this and looked forward to the second term to see how she was adjusting. While I appreciated the lovely facilities of the new daycare, I was unhappy with their lack of communication. There was a WhatsApp group, but that was for communication from them to us. It was mainly for announcements. I didn't know my daughter's teacher, and whenever I asked for her name or tried to meet her, she was never around. I preferred to speak with one person rather than the whole school, which is why I wanted the teacher's name.

Despite my ongoing concerns about her speech, I still hoped someone would tell me I was wrong, which they eventually did. One day, I received a letter from the school about a speech therapist assessment. I eagerly completed and submitted the form. After two weeks, I followed up to see if the assessment had been completed. They told me they would get back to me, but after another week had gone by, I was told that they had lost the form. By this time, my daughter was four years old, and I had promised myself that if her speech hadn't improved by then, I would seek help. Filling out that speech assessment form was my way of reaching out for support, and I was so disappointed that they had lost it and didn't even notice.

I realised I needed to take action instead of waiting for someone else to help. I started searching for speech therapists in my area. The first one I called charged R3,700, and they didn't accept medical aid. I was shocked. I don't know about you, but I certainly didn't have that type of money lying around. I couldn't understand why they wouldn't accept medical aid, as that was supposed to assist us in times of need.

After that, I kept searching until I found a therapist close to home who did accept medical aid, and their cash assessment fee was around R1,000. I booked an appointment and took my daughter. While all this was happening, I decided to withdraw her from her crèche as I felt she was not receiving the support I was paying for. I was looking for individual attention, and I didn't feel she was getting that. The detailed report they promised was also disappointing and not what I had hoped for.

2

My Worst Fears Confirmed

In September 2022, we finally attended our appointment with the speech therapist. One thing about my daughter is that she is fearless; she is not afraid of the dark, heights, or anything. However, as we entered the doctor's room, she started crying, and honestly, I wanted to join her. I knew that our lives would never be the same after that appointment, whether for the good or the bad.

When we met the doctor, her first question after greeting us was, "Who referred you?" I explained that it was a self-referral based on my observations, as I wanted to know the truth. I was tired of wondering if she needed help or not.

The doctor conducted a few tests, asking her questions, and I had to stop myself from crying throughout the exam. It is one thing to hear your child struggling to articulate herself in her safe home environment; it is another thing entirely when it happens in a professional setting. My heart broke for her during the assessment.

At the end, the doctor said what I had always suspected yet feared: my daughter had a speech delay. Her articulation of certain words was not appropriate for her age, and her speech should have been clearer by now.

Though I suspected it, hearing it confirmed was absolutely painful. I did not feel the relief I had anticipated; instead, I felt overwhelmed. The doctor recommended that we see her once a month, encourage her to use her words more instead of pointing at things, use the language she would encounter at school—English for us—and practice the words with her. After the appointment, we went to buy her ice cream, but all I wanted to do was get home and cry.

In that moment, I missed my late mom so much, or her late great-grandmother, who passed away in 2021. You might wonder why I needed them; I knew they couldn't fix anything, but I wanted them to hold space for me as their child, not as a mom. As a mother, I needed to be strong for her, to provide guidance and stability for our family. Yet, as Joey, all I wanted to do was cry and not stop. Suspecting that something was wrong and having it confirmed was heartbreaking. As much as I thought I was ready for this, I really wasn't. Can anyone ever truly be ready for such news?

Like any normal human being, I began to wonder if maybe I should have sought help earlier. Perhaps I had waited too long. Why had I not trusted my instincts? Fortunately, or unfortunately—depending on your context—we live in a world that now embraces the idea that kids are different and that their milestones are unique to them.

Therefore, I did not rely on my previous experiences with her brothers; I didn't want to compare her to them.

Based on my experience, my advice to you is this: **if you are uncomfortable with any aspect of your child's development, seek help.** It is better to be the mom who overreacts than the one who regrets her decision later. It is never too late to seek assistance. You can start today; as you read this book, pause for a moment and book that appointment.

We informed her brothers of her diagnosis and asked them to assist us. We spoke to our loved ones so they would know how to interact with her as we embarked on this new journey. My first concern was that I didn't want her to feel that something was wrong with her. The plan was to do the exercises with her in a fun and consistent way. There was no time to think about my feelings; I needed to focus on giving her the support she needed. I do not recommend this strategy, but realistically, most of us will be in fight-or-flight mode.

Now That We Have a Name, What's Next?

It turns out that being consistent is not easy, even with important things—who would have thought? Now that I had a name for what was happening, I began searching for a daycare for her. I wanted one that would not treat my child like a number because she is not one. With a referral from a friend, I found a daycare, and when I went for the interview, I truly connected with the owner/principal. Based on my previous experience, I was not taking any chances this time; I asked questions relevant to our situation and informed her that my daughter has a speech delay. I did not want any misunderstandings, and I realised that this time I was not willing to "keep the peace" or suppress my feelings only to regret it later.

The principal explained that they had previously worked with kids with speech delays and collaborated with a speech therapist who attended to them at their centre. I was happy with the school, and we officially started our journey with them in October 2022. I loved how they communicated with us; they sent updates during the day about what they were doing, and I could see that my daughter was receiving the attention she needed to blossom. For the first time, I could hear her singing songs—something she hadn't done at her previous daycare. This might seem like a small detail, but please pay attention to the little signs; they will indicate whether your child is receiving the necessary support.

At home, we continued with the exercises, which honestly were quite triggering for me. She still struggled to say words that seemed so simple to me, and it was heartbreaking to see that she genuinely thought she was saying them correctly. I looked up YouTube videos and articles on how to assist her, but they left me feeling even more discouraged. In October, we went for our second session with the therapist. I told her that I felt my daughter didn't know how to control her tongue. She suggested some exercises for her to practice. At the end of the session, my daughter was in tears from exhaustion. Sadly, there was nothing I could do but comfort her, then cry when I got home. I was just tired of going through challenges, and this one hit harder. Seeing your child struggle and be in pain is difficult, and knowing there is no instant solution makes it worse.

I remember attending the "Life Designed by Her" Masterclass hosted by Leanne Dlamini, where I shared my daughter's diagnosis. It wasn't my plan to share, as I was extra careful about whom I confided in when it involved my child. However, I was surrounded by love, and I thank God for that supportive space.

One thing I sadly realised early in our journey was that there was not enough support for families. You receive a life-altering diagnosis without any practical support on how to cope emotionally. The expectation is for you to continue living as if nothing has really changed, but for you, it has. Most of us don't have the tools to navigate such a diagnosis. No parent plans for their child to be sick or to be different from other kids; when it happens, it feels unfair to expect parents to carry on as if it is business as usual because it is not. Even if the child eventually turns out fine, it doesn't minimise the impact or toll that the process of getting there will take on the family.

One of the decisions I had to make early on was to accept the reality of my situation—that this was painful and hard. I am not going to pretend it is easy because it is not. That is why I decided to contact a therapist from work; I could see that I was on autopilot. I was showing up for my family, doing exercises with my daughter while also working my nine-to-five job. On the outside, it seemed that I was coping or making the best of the situation; however, inside, I knew that I needed help before I crashed.

If you are going through something similar, this is my encouragement to you: **it is okay to seek help. It is okay to feel**

overwhelmed. It is okay to feel that this sucks. It is okay to ask why this is happening to you or your child. It is okay to mourn the loss of what could have been. This does not mean that you do not love the child you have; it simply means you are accepting that this is not easy, and we should not romanticise it. Even if some good eventually comes from it, this is not the ideal situation, and most of us would not choose this journey, especially for our kids.

3

You Are Allowed to Change Your Mind

One of the things I have observed as an adult while raising my kids is that I have somehow lost the courage to change my mind—the courage to choose differently. I believe this is not unique to me; I have seen many people stay in situations that are no longer working for them, either because they are overly concerned about how others will react or because they are afraid to admit they made a wrong decision.

While checking my daughter's progress at school, her teacher informed me that, although she is able to communicate her needs, she felt that my daughter's speech improvement was slow. She asked if I could consult the speech therapist to recommend which areas we should focus on. Her question made me realise that I was not 100% happy with our current speech therapist. It wasn't personal; I just felt she wasn't the right fit for us. While she was great, she was not what we needed. I required someone who could guide us or provide templates to use.

With the current therapist, it felt as if, due to her previous experience with other patients, she took our situation lightly. For us, this was a new experience, and it was scary and overwhelming. I would leave our sessions feeling like I needed more information, which often led me to use Google to answer some of my questions. I do not recommend this because much of the information available is unverified and requires a professional's insight. I hated that I needed to conduct my own research; I can't be both a mother and a therapist to my child.

My daughter struggled with sounds; for instance, she would say "d" instead of "g" and "t" instead of "c." While this may seem simple to articulate, it was a challenge for her. I watched YouTube channels for tips—some worked, while others didn't. I felt our speech therapist should have shown us how to approach these challenges.

Based on her teacher's feedback, I contacted the therapist from her daycare. Before doing that, I read her reviews, which were impressive. When I phoned her, she was warm yet professional, and I felt a connection with her. She then sent me assessment forms to complete, which were thorough and asked about my journey from pregnancy to the present. This felt like exactly what I was looking for.

As a Black woman taught not to offend others or shake things up, even when I am unhappy, changing my speech therapist felt wrong and uncomfortable. Despite knowing it was for the best, I decided to set aside my discomfort and prioritise my daughter's needs.

Let's Try Again

As a side note, one of the ongoing lessons I'm learning as a parent is the importance of fighting for my kids, even when it makes others uncomfortable. The truth is, no one else will advocate for them as we do.

So, we went for an assessment with the new therapist, and she provided a detailed report recommending that we meet four times a month. She also suggested additional exercises and advised that my daughter undergo a hearing test. She recommended two audiologists—one didn't accept medical aid and had an exorbitant cash price, while the other accepted medical aid and had a more reasonable cash price.

On 9 December 2022, we went to the audiologist. She was very friendly and professional, asking detailed questions about my pregnancy, birth, and my daughter's early years. My daughter had only undergone one hearing test when she was born, and I now wonder if that was enough. We mentioned that she doesn't like her ears being touched. Even during bath time, she feels uncomfortable when we clean them. She doesn't cry or react drastically, but her body language and verbal cues make it clear that she dislikes it.

The audiologist performed a test and found that my daughter had a middle ear infection in her left ear, which caused temporary hearing loss. That's when it clicked—maybe this is why she struggles to articulate certain words: because she couldn't hear them clearly. As I had mentioned before, she often had a runny nose after starting daycare, but it wasn't severe, and she always improved with medication. We learned to manage it, ensuring she wore socks indoors if she wasn't wearing shoes.

Listening to the audiologist's explanation made everything make sense. My daughter had been dealing with a runny nose for over two years at daycare. Could this have been affecting her speech all along? The audiologist referred us to an ENT specialist to examine her further and recommend treatment. We'd need to return for another hearing test afterward.

While I was there, I realised how much information is not readily shared with us as parents, especially when it comes to specialists. Most of us only see them if referred by a GP, but what happens if the GP doesn't notice what you're seeing as a parent? I'm learning that it's okay to refer yourself, but the reality in South Africa is that many people relying on public healthcare don't have that option. I left the session with mixed emotions—relieved that we had finally discovered what was wrong but saddened that we didn't know sooner. I also felt guilty for not trusting my instincts earlier.

4

Toxic Positivity

Since I heard the diagnosis, I don't think I've truly felt thankful. Yes, I was grateful that we had the resources to offer her the help that she needed and that the diagnosis wasn't severe. But I was still angry that we were going through this in the first place. Throughout all my pregnancies, I prayed for my unborn children to be healthy, to reach their milestones—just like any other parent. Before this experience, it seemed that all my prayers were answered. My kids hardly ever got sick, and if they did, it was just a mild flu that would pass quickly. I have always been so grateful for their good health, fully aware that this wasn't the reality for many other families.

As a Christian, I have always been honest with the Lord about how I felt. Over time, I decided not to normalise struggle and pain as something that comes from God. I couldn't worship a God who brought suffering just to prove His power. For me, pain, sickness, suffering, and death are part of this broken, sinful world—but not God's perfect will for us.

When we received the diagnosis, I went back to my Heavenly Father and cried. I didn't sugarcoat it. I told Him that I hated what was happening. I expressed that I was tired of fighting, of being strong. I wanted ease, and this was not what I had asked for. Earlier in the year, I had lost my aunt—my late mother's youngest sister—leaving behind four young children. I was still processing that loss. Just ten months before that, I lost my grandmother-in-law, my confidante, and while grieving her, we lost Malome, one of our family's pillars. So, trust me when I say I didn't want to be tested. I didn't want to be made stronger. I just wanted to be held. I wanted my baby to be okay and not to have to go through this struggle.

Most importantly, I didn't want to hear that this was God's will for us or that He had chosen her for this because, honestly, why her? Since that day, I haven't been able to pray the way I used to. My prayers became tears, or sometimes I would just sing worship or praise songs with tears in my eyes. I didn't know how to fight this one, but I knew the only way I could survive was by continuing to believe in God's goodness despite it all.

One thing I kept reminding myself was that God loves my daughter even more than I do. He has already fought for her. He knew her before she was formed in my womb—before my husband and I even thought about having her. The Lord already knew she was coming. I would say these things softly in prayer or silently in my heart while doing other tasks. I decided that I didn't believe this situation came from Him, but I also believed that He could work it together for her good. I wasn't sure how, but I had to trust that all this pain would make sense eventually. We couldn't go through this for nothing. There had to be a bigger purpose behind it all.

If you're going through something like this, I hope you know that the Lord can handle your honesty. He can handle your "why me?" questions and your fears. No, He hasn't given us a spirit of fear, but fear is part of this fallen world, and He understands that. I remember a sermon at our church by Reverend Ralekgolela titled "So That." He shared the verses from John 9:2-4 about a man born blind. The disciples asked who had sinned, the man or his parents. Jesus responded that no one had sinned, but that it happened so that the works of God might be displayed in him.

That message was freeing for me. While I knew my daughter's diagnosis wasn't my fault, I had been carrying thoughts like, "Maybe I could have done something sooner," or "Maybe I should have been more proactive and trusted my instincts." But that morning, I was reminded that it wasn't my fault—and that God can use this for my daughter's good.

On 13 December 2022, we went to see the ENT specialist at the hospital. Before we even reached the doctor's office, my daughter had already decided she was done. She told me, "I'm not sick," meaning she didn't see why she needed to see the doctor. Honestly, I understood her—she didn't seem visibly ill, and I wasn't even sure how to describe her diagnosis. To tell you the truth, I didn't want to go either. I just wanted everything to return to normal, but it wasn't.

After filling out the forms, we finally saw the doctor, but he couldn't perform a full examination because, as I mentioned, my daughter has always disliked having her ears touched, and today was no different. After some persuasion, she allowed him to examine her ears, although it wasn't as thorough as he would have liked.

Can we talk about how challenging it is to navigate your child's discomfort or fears while also knowing that you'll be billed for seeing the doctor, regardless of whether the full tests were completed? It's not about blaming the professionals—they deserve every penny they charge because of their years of education, training, and expertise. As the saying goes, "If I do a job in 30 minutes, it's because I spent 10 years learning how to do it in 30 minutes. You owe me for the years, not the minutes." Doctors dedicate themselves to their craft, and their skill is invaluable.

But that doesn't change the reality that, for many parents, financial worries add to the emotional strain. **We can respect the expertise of medical professionals while acknowledging that the costs of healthcare can be a burden for families.** It's not about shaming either side—professionals for charging their rates or parents for worrying about finances. The truth is, many of us are doing our best with limited resources, trying to balance both the wellbeing of our children and the realities of our financial situation.

This was the added burden I was facing. There are so many emotions to navigate in such a short span of time. Watching my daughter squirm in discomfort, knowing I would have to bear the financial cost for something that was causing her pain, brought an overwhelming sense of frustration. I found myself feeling resentful—not only toward the situation but also toward the system—the doctors, the institutions. Yet, at the same time, I knew I had to be grateful that I was even able to bring her here and get the help she needed, help that I wasn't in a position to give her myself.

It's a difficult balance to strike—being thankful for access to healthcare while feeling the weight of financial strain. I had to remind myself that there are children who will never have access to even the limited resources I can provide for my daughter. But still, that sense of unfairness lingered. Why did we have to be here at all? Why was my daughter going through this when she shouldn't have to?

Bringing myself back to the consultation, I mentioned to the doctor that I felt she struggled with controlling her tongue. Despite the challenge of her not fully cooperating, he tried to check it. I really respect doctors who work with children—it requires immense patience. That's one of the key lessons I learned on this journey: as a parent, you must notice everything, even things that may seem insignificant. If possible, keep a small notebook to jot down the details you observe about your child. These might become important points to raise with the doctor later. **After all, you are the expert on your child.** You've been raising them, and there are things the doctor might not pick up in the limited time they spend together, especially when your child may not feel comfortable during the consultation. It's best to go in prepared with questions and concerns.

It's okay to be the mum who seems to know too much or who asks a lot of questions. This is about your child, and we can't afford to take chances. People will adjust. Growing up, especially as a Black woman, I was taught not to ask too many questions or talk too much, but motherhood has taught me otherwise—no one will advocate for my children except me. We need to unlearn those lies. **Your voice matters, Mama.** Speak up, even when your voice is shaking, even when your stomach is knotted with anxiety.

At the end of the consultation, the doctor finally confirmed that her tongue was tied, though it wasn't an obvious case—it was deep within. Someone finally heard me and validated what I had been trying to express all along. It was such a relief. She also had fluids in her ears that needed to be addressed, and her ear canal was small. Surgery was scheduled for January 2023. It was such a mix of emotions. I was relieved that the surgery would help her, but at the same time, I wasn't happy that she needed surgery in the first place. That's the duality of life.

5

Living While Waiting for Life-Changing Surgery

I tried so hard to focus on the present rather than the impending surgery. I wanted my daughter to enjoy herself as much as possible before January arrived. She loved swimming, and one of the things the doctor mentioned was that she wouldn't be able to swim immediately after surgery. So, my mission had been to let her enjoy it before everything changed.

Honestly, I kept praying for a miracle—for the doctor to turn around and say she no longer needed the surgery. But then, as soon as I had that thought, I felt guilty. Shouldn't I have been grateful that we finally had a plan, a solution that could help her? While I felt relieved that there was a possible resolution, the mother in me still wished it had been less invasive. I wanted it to be something as simple as a course of medication—just a few drops in her ears—

rather than surgery. At the same time, I wanted it all to be over, and I prayed that the surgery would be the permanent fix she needed.

One thought that carried me through was: "Two things can be true." I could give my children a joyous holiday season while still grieving inside. "Grieving" might have seemed like a strong word for what I was going through, but that was exactly what it felt like. I was grieving for what could have been, for the normality I wished for her. Outwardly, I might have seemed okay, and some days I even convinced myself that I was. But then I'd see my face in the mirror—the breakouts on my forehead, a telltale sign of stress. The last time I experienced this was in 2011 when I lost my mother, although the breakouts didn't start until 2012, because I never truly gave myself time to grieve.

In that situation, I did what was expected: I went into solution mode. Her long illness made me feel selfish for wanting her to stay. It didn't make much sense, but that was how society often pressured us into normalising death by shaming those who grieved into moving on quickly. I saw it in how I'd break down in tears whenever someone gave me the space to be honest about my feelings. It didn't matter if I was talking face-to-face or communicating via text—the tears would come. I constantly thought about my daughter, wishing she didn't have to go through this surgery in the first place.

As I reflected on this, I realised I had been moving through the five stages of grief, as described by Elisabeth Kübler-Ross. Even though this model was originally about terminal illness, it resonated with me. For many parents, receiving a diagnosis for their child felt like a life sentence—something to grieve, whether temporary or long-lasting.

This brought me to a question: why wasn't counselling mandatory for all families when they received a diagnosis, regardless of the outcome? The emotional toll was significant, and many parents—myself included—didn't even realise the depth of their feelings or that they needed support until much later. It shouldn't be left to parents to decide whether they needed emotional support or not. From the moment of that first diagnosis, psychosocial support should be available.

Please remember, these stages of grief aren't linear. Everyone's process is different. There is no formula, just insights into how others have navigated similar experiences. I hoped this model would help others process and articulate some of their emotions, giving them clarity on where they were mentally. I shared it from a place of empathy, as that had been my journey too.

1. **Denial** – In the beginning, there's the denial of the loss that has occurred. Life can suddenly feel meaningless, and we experience shock and numbness as the body and mind can only process so much at once. As the shock starts to wear off, more emotions gradually surface, and the weight of reality sets in.

2. **Anger** – Once we begin processing our loss, anger often emerges. It's a natural response, directed at the unfairness of life, at ourselves, or even at others. I remember being furious that my daughter had to go through this ordeal. I even asked myself, "Doesn't the devil get tired of attacking

40

me?" But attacking my kids felt like an entirely new level of cruelty. I was angry that help wasn't easily available— not just for me, but for others too. I felt enraged by a system that seemed to prioritise money over my daughter's health.

3. **Bargaining.** – This stage brings about the longing for life before the loss, a desire to return to how things used to be. I found myself wondering if things would have been different if we hadn't sent her to that first creche. Would she have avoided the ear infections altogether? Before we had her, my husband and I had decided we were done having kids, but as time passed, the thought of expanding our family grew on us. Eventually, we decided to have another child, and I thanked God that He gave us her. My husband always wanted a baby girl from the beginning, and now he finally had his princess. Gogo had been asking for a girl, too, so we were all overjoyed.

I wasn't particularly fixated on her gender—all I wanted was a healthy, happy baby. That's all. Yet, as we navigated this painful experience, my husband began blaming himself, thinking that because he had wanted her, she was now suffering. It broke my heart to see him feel that way, but this is what grief and pain do—they make us question everything.

4. **Depression**– While bargaining is focused on the past, depression focuses on the present. This stage is about grieving your loss without minimising your emotions. Sometimes, grieving with kids can feel like an impossible task—just as you begin crying, someone comes in asking

for bread, or someone else needs to use the toilet. The point is, you still need to find time to feel your emotions, even though life keeps pulling you back to the demands of daily life. As hard as it is, crying and feeling are part of the process.

5. **Acceptance** – Acceptance isn't about "moving on." It's about learning how to live with the loss. You adjust, but the loss remains with you in new ways. As I'm writing this on 30th December 2022, I haven't reached this stage yet. Right now, I'm just doing what I can to get through each day. Perhaps I'll revisit this chapter later and share how I feel once I've reached a place of acceptance. If you've already found ways to accept your loved one's diagnosis, I celebrate you. For those still in the midst of processing the news, I send you love and prayers. Remember, your grieving process is unique to you and your family. There is no right or wrong way to feel.

6

New Year, New Hope

By the third day of the new year, I found myself feeling hopeful. After enduring a period of fear, pain, and despair, I began to notice a shift in my emotions. Instead of viewing my daughter's surgery as something negative, I started to see it as a potential long-lasting solution. A friend helped me see things differently when she reminded me that God often uses physical means to perform His miracles. I started to embrace the idea that this surgery could be the physical tool through which He would work a miracle for my daughter.

This experience has taught me that all feelings, no matter how overwhelming or contradictory, are necessary and valid. Just a few days ago, I couldn't hold back the tears, and the fear seemed all-consuming. But today, I felt different—more hopeful, less afraid.

A few days ago, I tried to book the surgery, which now requires an online process. I struggled with it—perhaps because emotionally, I was at my limit. The process didn't feel user-friendly to me, and I wished I could just go to the hospital and book it in person. We sometimes underestimate the comfort that comes from speaking to another human being instead of navigating impersonal systems. It took me three days to finally register, and I kept thinking about those who aren't as tech-savvy or those who don't have access to the internet. What happens to them? Are they not part of the system's target market?

My daughter's diagnosis has opened my eyes to many gaps in our healthcare and administrative systems. It has also made me more aware of the privileges I have compared to many others in South Africa. This journey has been eye-opening, and though it's challenging, I am beginning to embrace the hope and strength I need to move forward.

Myths and Beliefs

Growing up, I often felt shame and sometimes faced punishment for asking questions about disabled individuals. Adults seemed uncomfortable with the topic and preferred to act as if nothing were happening. When encountering someone with a disability, we were expected to pretend they didn't exist.

Recently, I shared with an elder in my family about my daughter's upcoming surgery. After wishing me well, she asked what kind of surgery my daughter would have, and that's when things became awkward for me. She began to recount how she had difficulty hearing in one ear and mentioned that one of our great-grandfathers also suffered from hearing loss. It didn't stop there; she further explained that one of our cousins had the same issue. It seemed like a family trait, with some of us inheriting it.

At that moment, I firmly told her that I refused to accept this information as a familial physical trait because I believed it could hinder how my daughter lived her life. If my daughter had been born with this condition and the doctor had informed us that there was nothing they could do about it, I might have felt differently. However, that was not the case. She could sense my irritation and quickly reassured me that she was just sharing her experiences. I ended the call and took a moment to calm myself. While I understood that she likely meant to comfort me, her words had the opposite effect.

I choose to maintain my faith and look forward to the surgery as a means to help my daughter. I am sharing this experience so you won't be surprised when different people try to offer explanations for what is happening with your child. Many of these explanations will not be medically or spiritually sound. You have every right to dismiss what they say as the final truth. Instead, do your own research and find what resonates with you. Your journey is uniquely yours, and you are the expert on your child's needs.

You Are Not Alone: Hope and Courage from Another Mother's Journey

Boingotlo Gill, Mom of M, 15 Years Old

What is your child's diagnosis, and how old were they when they were first diagnosed?

"M has been diagnosed with cerebral palsy and moderate hemiplegia, as well as Autism Spectrum Disorder."

What led you to seek the diagnosis?

"There was a noticeable delay in several expected developmental milestones, such as sitting up and rolling over. Initially, I brushed these off as typical for a premature child (I gave birth at 26 weeks). However, when he started crawling, I noticed some unusual behaviours that raised concerns. Unlike typical crawling, he would slither and pull himself up using only the left side, with his right hand often clenched in a fist and his right leg weaker than the left when he eventually began to walk.

After an MRI scan and several tests, he was diagnosed with cerebral palsy and moderate hemiplegia just before his second birthday. I had suspected he might also be autistic before the formal diagnosis;

46

his behaviours, such as meticulously arranging his toys without playing with them and having extreme reactions to sensory inputs, led me to Google, which prepared me mentally for what I might be facing. He was diagnosed with autism by a specialist shortly before he turned five. His sensitivity to sound, food textures, clothing textures, and certain smells was challenging, yet I've learned to manage these aspects over time, making adjustments in our outings to avoid busier environments.

By 20 months, he wasn't saying as many words as other children his age. When his speech began to improve, it mostly consisted of echoing the words we would say."

Did you immediately go to the doctor when you suspected that there was something "wrong"? If not, what hindered you?

"Yes, I did seek medical help, and I'm grateful for that decision as it allowed me to understand him better and make informed choices for his care. We started different therapies early on, which made a significant difference."

How was your experience when you first went to the doctor? Were your child's issues attended to? Did you feel that they heard your concerns as a mom?

"I took him to a paediatrician I had known since his birth, which made me feel comfortable. We had developed a rapport during his three months in NICU, and even now, he still checks in on M whenever we see each other."

How is your support system?

"I receive tremendous support from my family, even though I live about two hours away from them. Their love has always been felt, and when M was younger, he would stay with them during school holidays, allowing me to recharge. I understand that you can't pour from an empty cup, and I found attending a few counselling sessions in the early stages to be immensely helpful.

I often say that M has been a blessing in my life. After he arrived, countless blessings poured in, and I truly appreciate all the help and support from those around us. It's true what they say: God will never give you more than you can handle, and He equips you to bear it.

The various therapies he has attended have been invaluable. I appreciate that they understand the need to change his speech therapist when he doesn't connect with someone."

What are some of your challenges?

"Our education system often lacks a specific and targeted approach for fully including learners with mental impairments.
There is a significant gap in the implementation of inclusive education in South Africa and a lack of teacher training.

Teachers frequently struggle to support learners with ASD in achieving reasonable educational outcomes. I've accepted that I am often seen as a "difficult" mom because I continually advocate for my child, believing our education system fails kids with mental impairments. My focus is on engaging children with autism rather than solely prioritising academic outcomes, which can be frustrating for everyone involved.

Raising an autistic child comes with anxiety, especially when they cannot communicate their needs and wants. Trusting someone else to care for my child is challenging, as I constantly worry about the "what ifs."

Unlike more spontaneous parents, M thrives on routine and familiarity, which means I have to prepare him for any new experiences. I've come to terms with the fact that I cannot simply apply for a job in any location without considering his needs, which impacts many daily decisions I make."

What are your wins?

"I am proud to see that M's condition is raising awareness about autism. I've taken on the role of teacher and advocate for him and for autism awareness in general. While many people may know about autism, they often don't understand it until they encounter it firsthand, which has become an educational opportunity for many."

What have you learned through this experience?

"Although the journey has been challenging, it has been incredibly rewarding. I've always believed that there is a silver lining in every difficult situation. My son has given me countless joyful memories and stories that can bring tears of laughter. Because of my experience with him, I feel I have become a better person.

This journey has helped me appreciate the small moments that come with parenting. I find joy in even the tiniest progress, like when his brother recently taught him how to tie his shoelaces. While he still struggles with coordination, seeing that progress brings immense joy amidst the challenges of raising him.

Previously, I was a perfectionist who preferred order and planning. Now, I've learned to accept that some things are beyond my control, and that's perfectly fine. I am not a failure for this. Accepting what I cannot control and letting go of minor concerns has been a significant blessing. There are aspects of my child's condition that I simply cannot change, and worrying about them is futile.

I love how he helps everyone who meets him see things—or even themselves—in a different light. You cannot encounter him without feeling warmth and affection. Though many autistic children may struggle with eye contact, he does not. It truly is a spectrum disorder; two children with the same diagnosis can exhibit vastly different behaviours and abilities. He enjoys talking to people and often becomes impatient when they don't understand him, insisting that they are the ones with the problem, as everyone around him comprehends his unique way of communicating."

Would you want to change this experience?

"Honestly, I doubt it."

8

Life Post-Surgery

You know that feeling when something seems too good to be true? That's how I feel right now. All I can say is that "relieved" doesn't quite capture my emotions. Hearing my daughter shout and scream fills me with such joy—it's music to my ears. Although she still struggles with some words, what matters is that I can hear her loud voice.

From New Year's Eve until 12th January, the day of her surgery, my constant confession was that there would be healing on the other side of the procedure; that she would be fully restored and speak fluently. As I write this, a thought creeps in: what if it doesn't happen? But I quickly dismiss it with faith. It seems unbelievable that we are already here; my loved ones and I were prepared for the worst, and now it feels amazing to simply breathe and celebrate that it wasn't as bad as we expected.

Reflecting on 12th January, the day everything changed for our family, I remember seeing my baby in that hospital gown, the fear in her little voice breaking my heart. I tried so hard to be brave for her, reassuring her that everything would be alright until the final moment when I had to leave her in the surgical room. I had to trust that she would be okay and that the doctors knew what they were doing. Most importantly, I knew that the Lord had already gone ahead of us.

The day before the surgery, I discovered that we would only be staying for half a day before being discharged. That news was such a relief; I wanted us to be in familiar surroundings after the surgery. To make the process more bearable for her, I brought her tablet, her favourite blanket, and her daddy came along with the router—because nothing comes between a toddler and her favourite shows. Having her tablet helped keep her occupied while we waited for the operation.

It's funny how, once we said she couldn't drink water after a certain time, she suddenly wanted it first thing in the morning—a rarity for her. I guess it's true that sometimes the heart wants what it can't have. She woke up at 5 am, desperate for water, but with some distractions, she managed to temporarily forget it. I allowed her to choose her outfit to lighten the mood, and, as expected, she chose her pink tutu. Honestly, her outfit helped me focus on the bright side instead of my fears.

The check-in process was smoother than the online pre-admission, and the nurses were kind, though my daughter was not having it. Throughout December and the weeks leading up to her surgery, I had been telling her about it as gently as I could. However, living it is a different story. She was reluctant to wear the hospital gown or the disposable nappy, but with some gentle persuasion, she finally complied.

We arrived at the hospital at 6:20 am, feeling nervous, thinking we would be done by 8 am. However, around 7 am, the nurse explained that they only start surgeries at 8 am and that they always begin with the youngest patient, a six-month-old baby, before my daughter. By 8 am, all of us were understandably hungry and thirsty, but she couldn't eat until after the surgery.

Finally, around 9 am, we went in. Holding her as the anaesthetist put her to sleep was incredibly hard, and leaving her in that room with the medical team was the toughest thing I had to do. I wished parents were not expected to hold their children in the theatre room. Once outside, I just wanted to cry; it felt so heavy. I said a silent prayer for her, trusting that everything would go well.

Thirty minutes later, the doctor came out and told me her tongue was tied deeper than he had first thought and that they had put grommets in her ears. They decided not to remove her tonsils, which relieved me, as the recovery process for that was daunting for a worried mother like me. When they brought her out a few minutes later, she seemed smaller than before, but I knew that was just my anxious mind playing tricks.

Once she woke up, the first thing she said was that she wasn't coming to the doctor again. I couldn't blame her! She watched her cartoons, and I tried to feed her oats, but she only wanted a bit. We faced a struggle waiting for her to pee so we could be discharged, and while waiting, she got out of bed and went to play outside. I was simply amazed and beyond grateful.

You might not understand how, throughout December, I had anticipated the worst-case scenario after learning about her surgery and reading everything I could about what to expect. I was prepared for her to be bedridden and attached to me, yet here she was— playful and fearless.

After what felt like an eternity, she finally peed, and we were able to go home. Once we arrived, she resumed playing as if nothing had happened. All my loved ones, who knew about the surgery, understandably expected the worst; they laughed when I told them she was fine and eating more than usual.

As I write, I remember the story of Sarah and how God brought her laughter when she finally had Isaac. That's how I feel now; after everything we've been through, I'm crying tears of joy because I can see progress, even if it may seem small.

For her treatment, the doctor advised me to gently move my hand in her mouth to ensure that her tongue doesn't reattach, as the body might mistake the surgery as a mistake. I need to do this twice a day.

At first, it was easy since I was at home with her, but as our days grew busier, I would sometimes miss the morning treatment because I had to leave early. Unfortunately, some people can get triggered and aren't able to help when I'm not around. As time passes, we see the progress and may forget to remain consistent with her treatment.

Finding the "Right" Daycare Post-Surgery

I think we don't talk enough about how emotionally and financially exhausting it is to look for a daycare for your child. When you add the fact that they have some delays, it becomes even more complicated. My criteria before the diagnosis were a crèche that was safe, nurturing, and offered a combination of education and entertainment. I didn't consider whether the crèche worked with speech therapists or occupational therapists.

As I write this, I remember how, with the boys, I used to look at the forms for eye tests and speech therapy as unnecessary (the privilege of not being affected). I remember saying that I wouldn't take my kids to a multiracial daycare before they spoke or were potty trained because I felt it wasn't necessary. I honestly believed that they would only provide a fancy environment that taught them English. This was my view until the diagnosis. As I mentioned earlier, my aha moment came while talking to a friend; she mentioned how she didn't mind spending more on daycare because she was paying for speech therapy and facilities that most of our crèches in the township or rural areas don't have access to. When she shared that, I realised that most of us treat crèches as babysitting facilities instead of environments that educate our kids.

So, as I looked for daycare this time, my criteria were different. I wasn't interested in a fancy place; I wanted to know that they genuinely care about my child and that she is not just another number. I wanted open communication between me and the teachers, a small class size, and assurance that they would work together with her speech therapist.

I started searching in January, with my first preference being a Montessori crèche since she had previously attended one, and I felt they were gentle with her. Am I the only one who is always shocked at the crèche fees? There was nothing less than R3,000 for half-day, excluding food. Whose idea was it to exclude food from crèches? It baffles me. Then the full-day ones are around R4,000 upwards. Maybe it's just me, but I really do not understand because it's not like they were providing free extra murals or even speech or occupational therapy. I could end up spending R10,000 monthly on one child. Is this realistic for most families?

January ended without me finding a crèche that met our criteria, including financial feasibility. Thank God for her speech therapist, who kept referring different crèches until we finally found one on 6th February. It was close to her brother's school, small, and very affordable. I was shocked at their prices. I explained to the principal that we were attending speech therapy, and she assured me that they would take good care of her. The night before she went to school, I was so nervous, hoping this was the right decision for her. However, seeing how happy she was reassured me that it was the right decision for now. Sometimes, in this journey, that is more than enough.

As she started her new crèche, she also began her speech therapy after the surgery. She was excited to receive homework to do at home, just like her brothers. I am trusting God for complete healing and praying that she will be surrounded by people who will help her reach her milestones.

What Happens When Mommy and Daddy Are Not Around

In our last session, her therapist recommended that for our next session she should come in alone. She wanted to see how the session would unfold without my presence.

Honestly, I felt partially relieved, as it wasn't easy for me to remain neutral during our sessions. Sometimes, my daughter wouldn't respond, or she would become emotional and withdraw. I found myself torn between comforting her, encouraging her to keep talking, or allowing her speech therapist to take the lead. So, when the therapist suggested they meet without me, I welcomed the idea. I felt my daughter had been a bit clingy and resistant when I was there.

Interestingly, the therapist noted that my daughter had been more independent during their first meeting, which I wasn't part of. I realised she was enjoying the comfort of having me around. To prepare her for this change, I started discussing with her that I wouldn't be present for her next session after their one-week break. When the time came, the plan was for her dad to take her, but since I was available, we ended up going together.

When we arrived, she was asleep while we waited for her session to begin. Fortunately, her therapist came out to fetch her, without any tears. After the session, we decided to treat her to ice cream. While we were out, I received a video from the therapist showing that the session was going well—what a relief! Afterward, the therapist informed me that everything had gone smoothly, and she didn't even have to use the reward system to motivate my daughter to participate. On the way home, my daughter told me she liked her teacher, which felt like a significant win.

We've been doing speech therapy for about six weeks now. While I can hear improvements in her articulation, I still wish she were fluent already. I understand that the process of unlearning is challenging, but I wish it were less difficult for her. I long for the day when this experience will transform into a testimony of what we overcame.

I've also noticed something striking lately. It seems like I'm hearing more stories of children with disabilities. It feels as though every child suddenly has some form of special need. There seem to be more discussions about kids with speech delays or autism. I recall four years ago, I had limited information on these topics. In conversation with a friend, we reflected on whether more children are being diagnosed with autism or if the stigma around such conditions is slowly fading, leading to more parents sharing their stories.

You are not alone, and I hope that this story reminds you to keep on fighting.

In our journey, it's important to remember that you are not alone. Each story shared is a testament to resilience and the strength to keep pushing forward. May this narrative inspire you to continue fighting for your child's growth and development, no matter the challenges you face. Together, we can find hope and encouragement in our experiences, reminding us that perseverance is key.

My Journey with J: A Mother's Perspective

My name is Tasmin Bota, and my son's name is J. He is a six-year-old boy who was diagnosed with mild hypotonic cerebral palsy at the age of four.

Seeking the Diagnosis

"J was born extremely prematurely at 28 weeks gestation, weighing just 1.080 kg at birth. I was acutely aware that his premature arrival would necessitate vigilance regarding his milestones. By the age of one, we were referred for occupational, speech, and physical therapy due to delays in crawling and walking. Unfortunately, these delays didn't seem to alarm the medical team, or if they did, it was never communicated to me.

As the Founder and Executive Director of Preemie Connect, I had access to resources and insights not readily available to others. Through my work with children who have cerebral palsy, I began to suspect that J might be affected as well.

Some signs that raised my concern included:

- The way he curved his hands.
- His low muscle tone, which made him extremely flexible and floppy.
- His struggle to hold a pencil correctly or engage in activities like running and jumping.
- Although he could walk, he needed assistance with climbing stairs.
- Chronic constipation, which hindered potty training, and difficulties with eating solid foods.
  Ultimately, I took him to a private paediatrician, and we left that consultation with a lengthy list of "issues." After a few follow-up appointments, we received his diagnosis."

Seeking Help

"Initially, we took a break from follow-up appointments because I felt we were "getting lost" in the system. I also became pregnant with a high-risk pregnancy and wanted to focus on my health and

J's development. However, when I noticed no improvement, I devised a plan and sought further assistance."

Experience with the Doctor

"The paediatrician I consulted came highly recommended after thorough research. From a clinical standpoint, he was excellent, but his bedside manner felt cold and clinical for a children's doctor. While my concerns were addressed, his initial attitude implied that I was merely a mother and not an expert. In such situations, I have to remind them of my extensive knowledge regarding prematurity and assert that I am the expert on my child."

Support System

"This aspect is quite tricky. Unfortunately, we have lost much of our support system over time. When J was initially born, we had an abundance of support, but as the years have passed, that has dwindled. Many people mistakenly believe that once you leave the hospital, the challenges of prematurity are behind you. Currently, our primary support consists of my husband and myself. We are fortunate that the preschool J attends has been an immense support. Having a team that understands his needs and works collaboratively is a game changer. This required significant research and interviews to find the right fit. Additionally, the relationships I've built along this journey have been invaluable."

Challenges Faced

"Finances are a major challenge. Raising a child with special needs can be costly, especially when considering private medical and educational expenses. We've been fortunate to access specialists and therapies through a government hospital, which has significantly reduced our costs. However, this will change in the coming year as J will exceed the age limit for government support, necessitating out-of-pocket expenses for therapies.

Additionally, juggling multiple children and managing appointments alone can be overwhelming. Emotionally, I am lucky to have a friend with a cerebral palsy diagnosis who provides invaluable support. She shares her experiences, offering perspective on what J may face in the future. However, not everyone is fortunate enough to have someone who understands their journey, which is why we started a special needs support group."

Celebrating Wins

"Receiving a diagnosis eliminated much of the uncertainty. I wanted clarity on what was wrong and how we could work together to address it. With the diagnosis in hand, we could collaborate with our team of therapists, doctors, and educators to establish goals and strategies. In the past year, we have witnessed remarkable progress, almost like night and day."

Lessons Learnt

"One important lesson I've learned is that your child is not defined by their diagnosis."

8

Reflections Four Months Post-Surgery

It has been a while since I last wrote. Recently, I attended an event hosted by Mrs. Boledi, where one mother shared her son's diagnosis. I couldn't help but cry through my makeup. While our diagnoses differ, I resonated with the fear of uncertainty and the challenges that new information can bring. When she spoke about the importance of provision and having resources, I could truly relate, as it is incredibly challenging to provide everything my child needs to function at their best. However, she also shared instances of how certain things came easily for her child due to their diagnosis. **Hearing this reminded me that good can emerge from pain and confusion, and that is worth focusing on.**

Every time I learn about another child navigating life with a diagnosis, my heart breaks for them. Yet, I celebrate the fact that today's parents are advocating for their children rather than hiding them away, which gives me hope for the future.

I made the choice to reach out to my daughter's speech therapist, expressing my frustration with the pace of her recovery. Though I noticed progress, I wished for quicker results—something we all desire as parents. During my Instagram live sessions, I noticed that many guests confidently stated their children's diagnoses, while I hesitated to label the mild speech delay. This uncertainty made me question if I was in denial about her condition.

To address my concerns, I asked the therapist, who kindly provided possible timelines for progress, which was incredibly encouraging to hear.

Fear of Hoping for the Best

I spoke to a friend of mine about how I often struggle to react when people comment on my daughter's progress. I've realised that I tend to **dismiss** these comments instead of fully acknowledging their significance. Perhaps it's because I'm afraid to hope, or I want everything to be resolved quickly.

The truth is, I do see the progress she's making. I see how confident she is; the girl talks all the time, and I love that for her. I hear the random words she uses that we didn't think she knew. Yet, I also hear the moments when she struggles to say a new word, and my heart sinks a little. In those instances, I find myself battling thoughts like, "Maybe the surgery didn't work," or "Am I in denial?" This is why I spoke to her therapist to gain clarity about her condition. I asked if it falls under a neurodiversity diagnosis. She explained that while my daughter's speech delay was not caused by a neurological issue, it still happened for reasons that remain unclear.

After that conversation, I cried because the waiting is overwhelming and can make you feel crazy. I often wonder if I am doing enough, or if I should be seeking more help. I fear that my hope might disadvantage my child, even as I completely trust the Lord for her healing. As one of my friends once said, "Sometimes God's miracle comes through the doctors, therapists, or diverse professionals who help your child." Healing doesn't always have to be a supernatural event; it can also be practical, such as taking her to the doctor, ensuring she takes her medicine, or doing her exercises.

A miracle can look like her therapist telling me that she will now hold sessions at my daughter's school instead of us having to travel to her practice. You might wonder why I'm so thrilled about this news. It means the school will be involved in her sessions, aligning their lessons with her therapist's focus. Plus, it eliminates the constant back-and-forth travelling that had been wearing us down.

Our Mondays used to be chaotic. I'd have to pick her up early from crèche, rush her to appointments, and then return to collect her brothers. It felt like an endless juggling act. Now, we've been able to streamline our routine, and to say I am grateful is an understatement.

On June 5, 2023, we began a new chapter with her receiving sessions directly at school instead of us having to travel. Her first session at crèche went smoothly, and the relief I felt was immense.

No more stressing over early pickups or adjusting our entire day around therapy. We could simply collect her in the afternoon as usual. She was brimming with excitement, proudly telling me how her teacher came to her school. Her enthusiasm was a huge comfort to me, knowing that she didn't feel singled out or different because she needed to see her speech teacher. Instead, she embraced it as something special.

To make things even better, her teacher worked closely with the school to ensure she got extra practice twice a week. It was like receiving a double blessing! I can't express enough gratitude for her speech teacher, who went above and beyond for my daughter and our family. I only wish that this kind of collaboration and support could be available to more children and their parents. It's moments like these that remind me of the old saying: it truly does take a village to raise a child.

It's a Birthday Celebration

On Tuesday, July 18, 2023, I found myself reflecting on the conversations we had with my daughter's speech therapist the night before. She shared that my daughter is doing great and that they expect to finish therapy by the end of October. We are now focusing on teaching her the "sh" and "ch" sounds. I'm torn about how to feel. Should I be excited that the therapy is almost over, or should I be worried that it won't be enough? I guess this is a time for me to lean into my faith, trusting that the Lord will complete what He started in her.

We will be celebrating her birthday on July 23, and I can hardly believe my baby is turning 5 years old. I wish I could gift her with an easier journey, but all I can do is be here for her. She has been asking to go to the playground, go on vacation, have cupcakes, and wear tutu skirts; the list goes on.

On July 23, 2023, I went to church with her big brother for the 7 am service, knowing it would be a jam-packed day. When we got home, the birthday girl was already awake and bubbling with excitement, finally ready to celebrate her special day. She had been asking about her birthday for weeks, especially since the rest of our family celebrates their birthdays at the beginning of the year while hers is at the end. Apparently, she even refused to eat soft porridge, insisting that she would only have cupcakes today.

As I read her birthday messages from loved ones, she eagerly asked, "Mama, I want to listen; they must speak." So, I requested voice notes instead of text messages, and listening to her respond and articulate herself was an emotional moment. Seeing her confidently express herself without my help was priceless and made our journey so far worthwhile.

A lot can happen in a year. Around this time in 2022, I was often in tears, fearful of what the new year would hold for her. My heart broke every day as I wished I could take her speech delay, tied tongue, and ear infections away—or even undergo the surgery for her. I couldn't imagine my baby enduring all of that at such a young age. Now, after speaking to many parents, I realise that some children go through far more challenging surgeries. As I mentioned earlier in this book, everyone's experience and feelings are valid.

At this time last year, I was trying to create beautiful memories for my children while emotionally preparing myself for the upcoming surgery. I felt less angry but still hoped and prayed for an instant miracle. You might be wondering why I'm reflecting on this. It's simply because, on December 19, 2023, my thoughts and feelings have shifted.

We are currently busy buying stationery and school uniforms for my daughter as she prepares to enter Grade R next year. A few weeks back, I spoke to Roxanne, and she asked me how I felt about my daughter going to Grade R. I honestly told her that I was excited and relieved for her, especially since there was a time I wasn't sure if that would even be an option. Yet, I still feel nervous. Will she cope in a big school?

I've chosen for all my kids to start Grade 1 in a big school, allowing them to be babies for a year longer. However, her speech therapist recommended that we start her at a school where she will continue to feel safe and secure, ensuring continuity. I understand her point; my daughter has faced so many disruptions, and she needs stability. So, she will be leaving her crèche and some friends to start a new school and make new friends. I won't lie; I have fears about how she will adjust to this new environment, but I'm praying and trusting that she will cope. It doesn't help that little Miss is no longer interested in doing her homework, so I must find creative ways to practice with her. Who can blame her? It does get tiring doing the same things repeatedly.

But as her mom, I see the results. My baby is so confident— sometimes a bit too confident! She talks to anyone she meets, whether she knows them or not. This is what I prayed for: to see her confidently being herself.

Understanding the Role of Paediatricians in Child Health

In trying to understand the role of paediatricians in child health, I had a conversation with Dr. Natasha and asked some questions that I believe will assist mothers like me who need these answers but may not know where to find them.

Dr Natasha Zechner – Paediatrician

What Do Paediatricians Do?

"Paediatricians are doctors who specialise in the care of children, ranging from newborns to adolescents. In addition to treating sick children, they focus on promoting healthy behaviours and preventing accidents and diseases. Paediatricians carefully monitor children's physical, social, and intellectual development, striving to identify problems early so that intervention can begin as soon as possible. Their ultimate aim is to assist children in staying healthy and thriving, working collaboratively with parents and caregivers to provide advice and support for day-to-day challenges. The ultimate goal is to ensure a happy, healthy child who functions well within the family unit and is able to learn and grow."

Can a Parent Refer Themselves, or Do They Need a Referral Letter?

"You do not need a referral letter to see a paediatrician. Anyone is welcome to book an appointment if they have concerns or would like to schedule a well-child visit."

What Should Parents Look for Before They Visit a Paediatrician?

"Growth and development occur rapidly during the first few years of life, making it challenging to provide broad guidelines that apply to each age and developmental stage. Routine screenings are essential for detecting challenges early, long before a problem becomes established.

Ideally, all newborn babies should be assessed by a paediatrician soon after birth. The paediatrician will conduct a thorough examination to exclude any abnormalities and may recommend further screening tests based on risk factors. Regular well-baby visits are also recommended at 6 weeks, 6 months, 1 year, and annually thereafter. If your baby was born prematurely or has a chronic condition, these visits may occur more frequently.

Apart from these visits, parents should consult a paediatrician whenever their child is unwell and not improving with simple home care or if they have any questions or concerns regarding their child's behaviour or development."

Advice for Moms Who Hesitate to Visit a Paediatrician

"Many mothers might feel apprehensive about visiting a paediatrician at the first sign of a problem, fearing they might appear paranoid or overreacting. However, as a mother, you spend more time observing and interacting with your baby in various settings. You are constantly monitoring their progress and comparing their skills with those of other children, putting you in a unique position to identify potential problems early.

If something concerns you, it's always better to have it checked out. Generally, the sooner a problem is identified, the easier it is to resolve. Even if the concern seems minor, a visit provides an opportunity for the doctor to assess your child's growth and milestones while offering general advice. Childhood is a period of exponential growth and advancement; a seemingly insignificant issue, if left unattended, can escalate into a major predicament that could affect your child now and in the future."

Advice for Parents of Children with Uncommon Medical Diagnoses

"Receiving the news that your child has a confirmed medical condition can be an emotional experience. You may feel relieved that your worries have been validated but also experience feelings of anger or guilt. These emotions are perfectly normal.

Parents often delay or avoid identifying a problem, hoping it will resolve itself. However, once a diagnosis is made, it becomes much easier to understand what to expect and to plan a path forward. This knowledge empowers you as a parent to take necessary steps to help your child.

A team of medical professionals is available to assist you, and your paediatrician can guide you through this process, ensuring you have the support you need."

9

A New Chapter: Big School

When we received her first-term report, I was quite anxious about it. I tried not to focus on it, but I had been eagerly waiting for this moment. Despite her therapist's reassurance that she shouldn't have any trouble in a mainstream school, a small voice in my head wondered if I was setting her up for failure.

I still have fears about how her speech delay might affect her, and I can't help but wonder if there might be more challenges ahead that we haven't yet seen. These thoughts often creep in while I'm trying to sleep, prompting me to send a quick prayer to God, declaring His healing over her.

Sometimes, I notice that she mixes up words when forming sentences. For instance, when she needs to say a long sentence, it takes her longer than it should. She often struggles with pronouns, mistakenly using "he" or "her" even when we gently correct her. It breaks my heart that she has to fight for skills that came so easily to her brothers and other kids. It feels unfair that she must struggle to accomplish basic tasks.

To be honest, we have not been keeping up with her speech homework as diligently as before. She simply doesn't want to do it, and I understand that it might bore her. However, I worry that if we don't practise, she could regress. So, whenever I find the time, I try to sneak in some exercises, even if they aren't from her assigned files. It feels like a never-ending journey, just manifesting in different ways.

When the school sent home forms for eye and ear tests, I completed them because I wanted confirmation that she is okay. The ear test confirmed that her hearing is fine, although she had excess wax in both ears. We are now waiting for the school holidays to take her for a check-up. Thankfully, her eye test came back clear, which I am grateful for.

As I write this, I am aware that other parents face even worse fears, and my heart breaks for them. So, when I received her report, it brought relief to my heart; she is doing well overall, with only a few areas to work on. I can handle that feedback.
We had also agreed with her therapist to schedule a review in February, so I think we will proceed with that to ensure we're providing her with the right support. I met her teacher today, who shared some areas for improvement, such as describing shapes and adding more colour to her drawings. Overall, she is pleased with my daughter's performance.

I shared with her that my daughter was diagnosed with a speech delay in 2022 and underwent surgery in 2023. The teacher mentioned that she prefers to get to know the child first before looking at their file. That really touched me because, unfortunately, some people may judge children based on labels or diagnoses, limiting what they believe they can achieve.

While I understand that not all parents may agree with my perspective, I want people to see my child for who she is, beyond her diagnosis. I recognise that we are fortunate that her challenges are not always visible, unlike many others who do not share the same privilege. After I mentioned her therapy, the teacher acknowledged that it would help her better support my daughter now that she understands what we are working on.

I am truly grateful to God that we can provide her with the support and help she needs.

You Are Not Alone: A Journey of Understanding and Support

My name is Ms. N, and my son, S, is 19 years old.

Early Diagnosis

"My son was diagnosed with Attention Deficit Disorder (ADD) at the age of five. This diagnosis began when I was called to the creche by the principal and teacher, who presented his daily work and showed me the achievements of his peers. They expressed concerns that indicated my son might need urgent attention for his academic challenges.

This marked the start of a long journey. An educational psychologist was recommended, and an assessment was conducted to determine the nature of his disorder. At that time, I was informed that he would need to attend a special school tailored to his academic needs. Since it was late to register him for Grade 1, we opted for a mainstream school with the understanding that he would repeat Grade 1.

In 2011, he restarted Grade 1 at Lantern Remedial School, where the recommended medication was administered. However, I was surprised when I was called to the school at the beginning of the second term and told he was not coping with their academic structure. The remedial officials suggested he would need to transfer to a school with Learners with Special Educational Needs (LSEN) classes. Thankfully, I spoke with the principal during my inquiries at Florida Primary School, where there was a space available for him, and he joined immediately.

The LSEN class offered basic Maths, basic English, and Basic Life Orientation until he reached 13 years old, at which point he transitioned to a technical high school for vocational training. He attended this school until he reached the school-leaving stage.

Throughout this period of school transitions, S attended various remedial therapies, including speech therapy, occupational therapy, and general remedial therapy. His longest stint was with the occupational therapist, who recommended a super-special private school for better monitoring and attention. Unfortunately, finances did not allow for private schooling, so we continued with the LSEN class at Florida Primary School."

Advocacy and Acceptance

"I commend myself for my resolve as a mother. I knew this experience wasn't unique; many parents face similar challenges. All I wanted was the best for my child. Ultimately, his happiness mattered most to me, and I refused to watch him struggle within a mainstream curriculum.

I was able to explain this situation to my family and friends, advocating for what was necessary to see S grow positively. Accepting our circumstances was essential, and their support grew as I shared my experiences, inspiring others to help their acquaintances in similar situations."

Navigating Challenges

"Honestly, there were not many challenges during S's schooling, except during high school when he used common transport with mainstream learners. They occasionally made nasty comments about Roodepark School, derogatorily known as the "school for slow learners." However, I found it easy to reassure him that he was, in fact, doing much better than those mainstream learners, as he was receiving vocational training alongside his studies. This positive perspective helped frame our entire experience."

Important Lessons Learned

"The key lesson I learned is the importance of taking action. Don't wait for a situation to worsen; when faced with challenges, seek help and act promptly. For some parents, accepting their children's academic challenges can be difficult, leading them to keep their kids in mainstream schools until it's too late. No parent wants to see their child struggle or feel stressed, as this can lead to depression and, in the worst cases, suicidal thoughts. I learned that life isn't always straightforward, and maintaining a positive mindset is crucial. Trusting in the Almighty for guidance, strength, and wisdom is essential, and with that, everything else tends to fall into place."

Gratitude for Support

"I am truly grateful for the unwavering support of my family, friends, and now my husband. Their presence made navigating this journey far easier, and I couldn't have done it without them by my side."

You Are Not Alone: A Journey with Autism

My name is Roxzanne Klassen, and my son, R, is a 4-year-old male.

Diagnosis

"R was diagnosed with Autism Spectrum Disorder (ASD) Level 3 (non-verbal) at the age of 3."

Reasons for Seeking Diagnosis

"I sought a diagnosis due to several concerning signs and symptoms I observed in R. He exhibited regressive language skills, was a picky eater, walked on his toes, licked objects, and avoided eye contact."

Initial Hesitation to Seek Help

"Initially, I did not go to the doctor right away. I conducted extensive research first. However, the financial burden associated with specialists and doctors hindered me from seeking help sooner."

First Visit to the Doctor

"My experience during the first visit to the doctor was disheartening. I felt that the doctor was not fully present, coming across as cold and unengaged. Instead of addressing my concerns, he simply referred us elsewhere and reiterated information I had already gathered through my own research."

Support System

"Fortunately, I have an amazing support system. It took time for everyone to adjust, but their understanding has been invaluable."

Challenges Faced

"Most of our challenges revolve around financial concerns, particularly regarding doctors, therapies, and finding affordable schooling that caters to my son's specific needs."

Celebrating Wins

"Despite the challenges, we have celebrated significant wins. R has reached milestones that we once thought were impossible. Seeing him smile and embrace life fully has been a profound joy."

Lessons Learned

"Through this experience, I have learned to be more tolerant and patient. I've realised that nothing is impossible and that sometimes, silence speaks volumes.

Thank you for allowing me to share our story. I hope it encourages others who may be on a similar journey."

10

Navigating Nerves and Expectations

It was 6 AM on Thursday, 2nd May 2024, and I found myself awake early, even though I wasn't going to work and my daughter wasn't heading off to school. You might have already guessed it— the reason I was awake at that hour was nerves. We had a meeting with her speech therapist later that day, and honestly, I wasn't sure what to expect.

The check-up was part of the routine we had agreed on last year after completing her sessions, but now that it was finally happening, I understandably had questions. What would the therapist say about her progress? Would she recommend that we perhaps start lessons again? The truth was, I wouldn't have minded that. As much as I tried to support my daughter on her journey, I sometimes wondered if I was doing enough. I wasn't a professional audiologist or speech therapist; I was just a mum who wanted what was best for her child.

There were a few areas where she struggled, particularly with using certain words. For example, she avoided using "she" in her sentences, often resorting to "her," which was incorrect. This challenge was magnified now that she attended a girls' school, where she needed to use "she" much more often than she wanted. I planned to mention this to her therapist and hoped for some helpful suggestions.

I had also spoken to her father about enrolling her in an extra-curricular activity that required more verbal interaction, aiming to build her confidence. I noticed that when she met new people, she tended to withdraw and revert to baby language, which was quite different from how she spoke around familiar faces. I was still searching for a suitable activity, and perhaps the speech therapist would have some recommendations.

As I typed, I couldn't help but wonder if this behaviour was normal for a 5-year-old. But because of her previous diagnosis, I found it hard to take it lightly. I wonder if you can relate; once our child has a diagnosis, everything becomes serious. We analysed every detail, even if we didn't want to, fearing we might make a mistake that could hinder our child's progress. It was a huge responsibility on top of the usual mom guilt.

When you have a child who is struggling, every decision feels monumental. My heart broke for parents who were grappling with similar challenges, questioning if their choices could negatively impact their children's progress, even when their intentions were good. I had read about treatment fatigue—how individuals on chronic medication often default not out of choice, but due to physical and emotional exhaustion. From the outside, it was easy to judge someone for stopping life-saving medicine simply because they felt tired.

On a smaller scale, I had noticed this fatigue in my daughter after we ceased formal sessions. Although we continued with activities at home, our frequency of practice dwindled from daily to sporadic sessions, eventually leading to me forcing it upon her. She found ways to dodge or delay until I simply forgot or became too busy with other things.

As a working mum of three, my evening time was limited. We only had two hours to cook supper, assist with homework, bath the kids, and bond before bedtime, so inevitably, some things fell through the cracks. As I approached the appointment, I couldn't shake the feeling of uncertainty—had I done enough for her? Was I doing enough to help her become the girl that the Lord had created her to be?

On days like that, I needed to trust my heart for her. I truly loved this girl, and I would continue to do everything in my power to help her reach and exceed her full potential. I hope that you, Mama, would also trust your heart for your child. Your love for them is powerful, and remind yourself that you are genuinely doing your best. I reflected on how far I had come from where I started.

Did I mention that she had done her very first show-and-tell two weeks earlier? When I saw the rubric and instructions, I felt they were expecting a lot from the kids in a short period. She needed to know the whole family's ages, our address, and my mobile number. But you know what? She proved me wrong. She memorised it all and did exceptionally well; she even remembered my mobile number!

This experience served as a reminder that our kids are capable. Sometimes, because of what we had been through, I found myself being overprotective. I recognised that I needed to work on this, as I didn't want to block her success out of fear or the desire to shield her from embarrassment.

This parenting gig was definitely not for the faint-hearted.

Early Morning Reflections: Navigating New Challenges

It was 3:26 AM on a Friday morning, and I couldn't sleep. I wasn't surprised, considering what we had heard during our appointment. Based on her assessment, the therapist recommended that my daughter see an occupational therapist to prepare for Grade 1. Honestly, I was taken aback; to me, she didn't seem to have any issues with her motor skills. My daughter often performed physical stunts that scared me a bit, especially on the jungle gym.

However, the therapist pointed out that the way she wrote words upside down or backwards was something that could be addressed by an occupational therapist. She also noted that my daughter couldn't spin and count at the same time or jump and count, which were skills she was expected to have. I won't even lie and say I had noticed this because I had never tried it. I knew she could jump and spin, but I hadn't thought to combine those activities with counting.

So, our next step was to book an assessment with an occupational therapist. Meanwhile, my daughter would have two sessions a month with Nazmeerah, as the therapist felt they only needed to work on minor issues for now—there was no need to meet weekly unless she saw something else that required attention. It turned out that this regression was quite normal for kids who had experienced a speech delay and were now starting school. As much as I understood all of this, a part of me really hated the fact that we were starting yet another thing. When we attended the appointment, I was aware that there were a few areas we needed to address, but I didn't expect to begin sessions with another professional. I really didn't see that coming, and it wasn't easy to process without feeling as if we were somehow going backwards instead of forwards.

Another thing the therapist mentioned was how my daughter was now using her diagnosis as a crutch, despite being fine. I had also noticed that when things became challenging, she would mention how sick she was or resort to baby talk, which defeated the purpose of helping her. At times, she would become teary. So, we now needed to work on her resilience. As a family, we had contributed to this situation. Her diagnosis had shocked us to the point where we allowed certain behaviours that we shouldn't have. We also inadvertently enabled some of her unhealthy coping mechanisms because we felt that life was unfair to her. Having to deal with a diagnosis, surgery, and speech therapy, she had to learn and unlearn things that came naturally to other kids. She had to put in extra effort for things that other children didn't even struggle with, which felt unfair.

However, I was learning that instead of complaining about our situation, we needed to make peace with it and empower her. We couldn't change what had happened, but we could support her and ensure that it didn't hinder her potential beyond how it had already affected her beginning. Sometimes, it felt easier said than done, but I knew our kids deserved it. We needed to try and fight for their sake.

The therapist also explained that I would need to be actively involved in her learning; I couldn't let her figure things out alone like other kids, and some things might take extra time for her to process. We agreed that she would give me exercises to do with my daughter to prepare her for Grade 1 next year. As I previously mentioned, they currently didn't have homework, so the exercises were a welcome resource for me as I actively wanted to help her.

I don't know where you are in your journey, but I wanted to remind you that all the decisions and actions we took on behalf of our kids were not in vain; we would see the results. I knew it felt like this diagnosis kept taking and taking, and as I always said, sadly, it had no idea that "we can do hard things." We would do the hard work of fighting for our kids to have a quality life.

As grateful as I was that we could afford these resources for her, my heart went out to all the parents who couldn't provide the same support for their children due to a lack of resources. I also felt for the adults who had not received the help they needed as kids, leading them to face the world sometimes with a diagnosis that could have been worked on. I was so sorry that we lived in a world where such resources were not accessible to everyone.

Thank you to those who fought despite all the odds against them. We see and celebrate your resilience.

Conversation with Social Worker – Disabilities: Bulelwa Mahura

To better assist parents who might be facing similar challenges, I had an insightful conversation with social worker, Bulelwa Mahura. Our conversation covered a broad range of topics that are crucial for families navigating the challenges of disabilities. Here are some of the key points from that discussion:

What do social workers with disabled patients do?

"It depends on who employs them: government, NPO, private hospital, or if they are self-employed.

General duties and responsibilities include:

- **Intake:** Meeting for the first time, determining needs, registering, or enrolling for services.
- **Research and sharing information.**
- **Counselling:** Coming to terms with the disability, processing grief, acceptance, and living with the disability.

Counselling is holistic. The focus is not solely on the disability but on how it impacts the different facets of a client's life, including family relationships, school/work, and medical care. It also serves as a reminder that the person with a disability is still a complete human being with needs, desires, dreams, and aspirations. The individual is a growing entity—spiritually, mentally, emotionally, socially, and physically—and these aspects must be addressed too.

- **Family support:** Building healthy and supportive relationships within the family structure.
- **Building a network of human and physical resources:** This includes therapists (occupational therapists, physiotherapists), doctors, special education experts for children, and facilities for recreation and other activities accessible to people with disabilities.
- **Referrals:** Connecting people with disabilities and their families to relevant service providers.
- **Practical considerations:** Assistive devices, accessing services and amenities, and financial implications.
- **Advocacy:** Helping make services available or accessible."

Do we need a referral to see a social worker working with disabled children or adults?

"No. However, you may be referred by another professional who is aware of the availability of social work services, typically in a hospital setting. Alternatively, you can conduct your own research to find such a service."

From the time you started working with disabled children to now, what are some of the challenges you have observed?

"Unfortunately, I have not seen enough progress regarding awareness, sensitivity, and accessibility.

Our society is not sufficiently knowledgeable about the different types of disabilities. Because we lack information, we are unaware and insensitive. As a result, people with disabilities and their caregivers not only face physical barriers but also social barriers.

The people who have knowledge are usually those directly affected by disability—those who have disabilities, their loved ones, caregivers, and service providers (specifically in the disability sector).

This should not be the case because disability is supposed to be mainstreamed. That's why we have the Department of Children, Women, and People with Disabilities.

Mainstreaming within social work means that every social worker should be able to provide basic interventions or refer individuals to appropriate service providers."

Taking into account the emotional toll that this journey takes, are there any resources available to support families?

"Yes, there are organisations that were started by individuals and families affected by disabilities who did not find the support they needed. These organisations aim to provide support for others. The type of support available depends on the organisation and the resources they have."

How can parents holistically take care of themselves and their other children while going through this journey?

"This journey requires parents to slow down and intentionally address the various aspects of their lives.

Start with yourself. Ensure that your cup is full so that you have the energy to give to the rest of the family. Take alone time. Engage in daily practices that ground you. Eat nourishing food to strengthen your immune system, exercise for mental and physical strength, get quality sleep, take care of your emotional health, pursue at least one interest outside of family, and build strong relationships outside the family.

Release the guilt associated with taking time for yourself.

Then, focus on building a strong relationship with your spouse. When the two of you have a healthy relationship, it becomes easier to navigate the journey together and bring the other children on board. Spend couple time—resolve problems, do fun things, take care of day-to-day responsibilities, and maintain friendship and intimacy.

If you are a single parent, cultivate strong relationships with extended family, neighbours, support groups, and professional supporters. Ask for help and lean on your support system.

Honest, open, and empathetic communication is key. Everyone must commit to creating a safe environment for open and honest conversations about what they are experiencing. This includes listening, validating each other's experiences and feelings, apologising when something hurtful is said or done, offering forgiveness, and practising patience, grace, flexibility, and understanding. Parents set the example.

Each parent should ideally have one-on-one time with each child regularly—find what works for you.

No one should be left out of the conversation. Everyone should be included in building a relationship with the family member with a disability. Find solutions together. Keep everyone informed. Navigate changes together by creating the space and time for it."

> Any encouragement or advice to parents whose children are going through a new diagnosis or an old one?

- "Prioritise self-care so that you have the energy to deal with challenges and care for those dependent on you. Fortify your spirit, mind, and body.
- Encourage your loved ones to take care of themselves too.
- Adopt a growth mindset. Ask yourself, "What can I learn from this? What is unique about our situation? In what

ways has this situation changed us? How can we contribute to the lives of others because of our situation? What strengths has our situation revealed—about our child, about ourselves as individuals, and as a family?"

- You can ask, "Why me?" because we have been conditioned to ask that (it is considered human nature, and perhaps it is). But also ask, "How is it serving me to ask, 'Why me'?"
    - If it's from a place of truly seeking to understand and find resolve, then ask.
    - But if it's from a place of self-pity, give it a time limit and move on.
- Take time to feel your feelings. Allow yourself the grace to adjust to the new situation and any time something new arises.
- Allow yourself to grieve what has been lost.
- Clarify your values and let them guide you.
- Believe that this is in your reality because you can handle it.
- You are still in control of certain aspects of your life—have fun, do what you love, pursue your interests. You can address the challenges while still enjoying your life."

11

A Painful Mother's Day

Today, I met with her teacher, and to my surprise, I was much calmer than I had been when I first received the invitation. It was likely because my focus was already on the news from her speech therapist and the upcoming appointment with her Occupational Therapist. I kept reminding myself that whatever her teacher had to tell me wouldn't be as painful as the news I had already received. We had gone through so much already and come out on the other side. Whatever was shared in the meeting, we would handle it. We would be okay. We would show up for her, just as we always had, and continue to do so.

After four days of worrying, it turned out that the meeting wasn't even about my daughter or her performance. Instead, it was about a WhatsApp status I had posted on my personal account, commenting on a fizzy drink that she enjoys at school. It wasn't even a negative status, yet somehow it caught the attention of the school, and they wanted to know if I was happy with their services. I couldn't believe I had gone through so much turmoil over the weekend for something so insignificant.

After we cleared things up, her teacher committed that in the future, she wouldn't schedule a meeting with such a long wait in between. The anxiety during that waiting period had been overwhelming, and if I had known what the meeting was about, I would have had a much better week and weekend.

I was so relieved to find out that the meeting wasn't about her or her performance, but rather a misunderstanding that was easily resolved. I am grateful for her teacher; she genuinely seems to care about the children and is committed to ensuring their well-being. During our conversation, I mentioned that I wasn't sure how to practically support her with her academics, as they haven't been given homework. Her teacher explained that they were focusing on laying a foundation and that homework would be introduced in the third term.

I have decided to start using flashcards to help her on her learning journey. I've even created my own, thanks to YouTube. I don't know about you, but I hate the feeling of not doing anything to help. I understand that sometimes my actions may not be effective, but it's a risk I'm willing to take. I'd rather try something than not try at all.

That being said, I also know there are seasons where you need to be still, to refrain from trying new things or seeking immediate solutions, and instead simply embrace the stillness. Sometimes, doing nothing is harder than taking action.

As I commemorated Mother's Day, I was still reeling from the feedback I had received from her OT assessment. Since I couldn't physically attend the session and didn't want to postpone it, I asked her therapist to send me a voice message instead. Thankfully, she did, but listening to those short audio clips outlining concerns about her eyesight, hands, posture, hearing, and so on, left me feeling completely overwhelmed. My heart ached for my daughter, knowing that once again, she would have to summon her resilience. She would have to learn, unlearn, and relearn new skills, and I couldn't help but compare how much easier her brothers' journeys had been.

I found myself crying on her behalf, wondering why she couldn't have had a similar experience to her siblings. I understood that sometimes there simply weren't any answers, but that didn't stop my heart from wondering and asking those questions. You might be curious as to whom I was addressing these questions—honestly, I brought them before my Heavenly Father during my moments of prayer or whenever the harsh reality of our situation came crashing down. In those tearful moments, I shared all my questions with Him, because the truth was that, as much as others might have tried to comfort me, most couldn't provide the answers or the peace I so desperately needed. Only the Lord could truly reassure me and heal my broken heart.

If you are going through a similar experience, I pray that you give yourself permission to break down sometimes, so that you can continue showing up for your child. I had a conversation with a close friend whose children had gone through OT as well. I spoke to four friends in total, and they all shared how much OT had helped their children, how it had improved their quality of life and supported their progress at school. One friend even told me how her four-year-old child had learned to write their name after OT sessions had helped them grasp a pencil correctly.

So, I reminded myself to focus on the brighter side—that even this difficult experience was ultimately working together for her good. It would enhance her life, even though the process itself was anything but pleasant. On this Mother's Day, it felt bittersweet. I longed for my mother, wishing she were here to hold my hand through this journey. I also couldn't shake the nagging feeling of wondering if I had done enough for her. Was there something I could have done earlier to protect her from this? Had I missed anything that could have made life easier for her from the start? I knew these questions weren't entirely rational, but I couldn't help myself.

I also knew that I wouldn't always feel this way, but at that moment, it was how I felt. If you are going through something similar, I pray that you are surrounded by people who remind you that, despite your child's diagnosis, you are still an amazing mother.

What Happens When The Experts' Diagnosis Doesn't Resonate With You?

It was the 15th of May, and I was feeling so much better after processing the OT's feedback. I was reminded again that, as much as she is an expert and a professional in her field, I am also an expert when it comes to my daughter. No, I wasn't in denial about what my daughter needed, which is why I sought help as soon as I suspected that something was amiss with her development. That's why I took her to a speech therapist without any referral, because I was not in denial. That's why, when I saw that she wasn't receiving the help I believed she needed, I sought a second opinion—proof that I was not in denial, but rather a mother who recognised her daughter needed help and was willing to do everything in her power to get it for her, including putting her through surgery and months of speech therapy.

I needed to remind myself of all this because, sometimes, the world can make you doubt your instincts and intentions, especially when they differ from what the experts say. As I listened to her OT's feedback, some of the points didn't align with what I know about my daughter. It made me wonder whether we sometimes expect too much from our children—expecting them to perform without nerves in front of complete strangers. Yes, the assessments are done in the form of play, but that doesn't change the fact that these children are left alone with a stranger, doing an assessment for the very first time.

I'm not here to judge whether this method is right or wrong, but I know that, as an adult, I don't always perform at my best around strangers, and I sometimes wish I could bring a familiar face with me. So, why do we expect young children not to feel the same way? Furthermore, my daughter is a black child, and English is our second or even third language, yet all these assessments are conducted in English. She is being evaluated from a Western perspective, rather than from the African reality that she lives in every day. Some of the words, shapes, and colours she is expected to know are things that, at 40 years old, I am only learning now while raising my children. Is it fair to assess all children using a Western, English-speaking standard?

Do we even consider that their daily experiences might be different? Many children do not have the same access to resources or opportunities as English-speaking children with privileged backgrounds. Some children don't have English bedtime routines, or regular visits to the zoo, planetariums, or theme parks until their schools organise such trips. The reality is that what might be considered normal for a child from a well-resourced background is not a norm for a child whose parents are still trying to make ends meet. These assessments should take that into account.

A trivial example: one of the words used for the letter "I" in the alphabet is "igloo." Honestly, how many people use that in daily conversation? I certainly don't. So if I, as the parent, don't use it, how can I expect my daughter to know it when I haven't exposed her to it? While processing the OT's feedback, I had to remind myself of my daughter's own realities—realities that the theory may not take into account. As I often say, theory is so much easier than reality; it doesn't account for the nuances of people's actual lives.

That said, there were points the OT mentioned that did resonate with my own experiences with my daughter. A close friend reminded me that, while professionals can provide insights, whatever they tell you should align, at least in part, with your own observations. It shouldn't feel completely foreign. For instance, even though I didn't have the medical term for my daughter's initial diagnosis, I was able to understand what the doctor was saying. I could even point out things I had observed during our day-to-day interactions—things the doctor might not have checked if I hadn't mentioned them. For example, her tongue being tied wouldn't have been examined had I not expressed concern, even though I wasn't sure what the problem was at first. Because of the information I shared, the doctor was able to investigate and recommend a solution.

As I continue on this journey, I've been reminded that it's okay to question some of the medical findings. I must trust my own knowledge of my daughter. I may not have medical qualifications, but I am qualified when it comes to understanding her needs, and I will fight for her. So, that's my current plan: to take one day at a time, listen to the experts, but seek clarity or even a second opinion when I feel it's necessary.

Speaking of second opinions, I must acknowledge that it's not as easy as it sounds. I don't know about you, but I don't have endless amounts of money to spend, so seeking another professional opinion is not always an option for me. With her speech therapy sessions starting soon, we don't have extra funds for another assessment right now. So, for now, I'll wait for our in-person feedback session.

Meeting The Occupational Therapist

I finally met my daughter's Occupational Therapist, and she was lovely and very kind. I continue to advocate for in-person meetings and feedback over written or virtual communications. Speaking to someone face-to-face felt different. We had a few minutes where I broke down, but I left the meeting feeling hopeful and empowered.

One important point the therapist made was that we often forgot how different the world was for our children compared to our own experiences. Most children her age and younger had spent two to three years of their lives during the pandemic, which significantly impacted their socialisation. Many could not go out to play or interact with other children or adults, affecting their physical development. They had more screen time and less physical activity, and I could sadly attest to that. As I had mentioned before, my daughter only attended daycare from the age of two; prior to that, she had been cared for by her late great-grandmother, who did her very best.

In addition to being affected by COVID, my daughter, unlike her brothers, did not play outside our house, and space within our yard was limited. This was a stark contrast to my own childhood, where we played in the streets, skipping, pretending, hiding, and playing with mud—activities that unknowingly prepared us for school. Unfortunately, for her and most of her peers, those experiences were lacking, which was why she needed occupational therapy to close that gap.

I was able to share some of my concerns and ask clarifying questions, which the therapist addressed. She also recommended swimming lessons or horse riding, and I was grateful that we could provide those opportunities for her. However, my heart could not help but wonder about the children whose parents could not afford such activities. Additionally, she suggested multivitamins, and they would have weekly lessons for the next six months. I left the session feeling less anxious and ready to do the work.

There was a moment when I wished I were a housewife so I could focus entirely on her, but at the same time, we needed the income to meet all her medical needs. So, once again, I had to trust that I was doing my very best, and that would have to be enough.

A Prayer of Forgiveness for a Mother with a Child Who Has Received a Diagnosis

Heavenly Father, thank You for revealing what is happening with my child. Though the news may not be what I expected, I am grateful that we now know what we are dealing with.

As we embark on this new journey, I pray for wisdom, peace, resources, and strength to navigate it. When self-criticism arises, may I remember that I deserve the grace I extend to others. Help me forgive myself for not noticing the signs or for not acting sooner when I suspected something might be wrong. May I let go of the guilt for any area I feel I could have handled differently.

Please guide me to be kind to myself, silencing the "what if" questions and the "if only" thoughts. Help me accept the realities of our current situation and focus on what I can control. I recognise there is only so much I can do as a human being, and that the rest is in Your hands.

Because You love my child, know them by name, and have good plans for them, may I hold on to this truth on days when things feel heavy. Thank You that even now, You are healing us as a family. In Jesus' name, Amen.

12

Maybe I'm Having A Pity Party

That was my thought today after I spoke to someone about what we were going through. When I complained about the expectations on kids, especially how westernised everything had become, she mentioned a truth that was hard for me to accept: the only reason I was complaining about the methods and content of learning was because my daughter was struggling. Although I wanted to deny it, she was right; the reason I noticed all these things was that I was personally affected. Perhaps other parents had gone through similar experiences before, and what I was facing might not have seemed like a big deal to them.

As much as I understood this, I was also aware that their experiences did not invalidate my feelings and observations. The fact that I was only noticing some of the gaps now did not negate my observations. You might have gone through a similar experience where, because of your child's diagnosis, you began doing your own research and started questioning things you had either not been interested in or had only been aware of because they didn't personally affect someone you knew. You might have accepted them as normal without probing deeper.

I am just here to say that this did not make you selfish or inconsiderate of others' challenges; it simply made you human. Trust me, you are not the only person to do that, and you would probably not be the last one. Honestly, I celebrate the fact that you were asking questions, whether to your family, friends, or the world at large.

As a disclaimer, she wasn't mean or anything like that; she was simply encouraging me to focus on my daughter's healing instead of wanting to change things that had always been there. Other kids learned the same content and did well, so perhaps the problem wasn't the method itself, but rather the fact that the method was standardised for all children without considering their individuality. This challenged me to reflect again on whether I was in denial about my daughter's situation. After sitting with this question, I realised that I was not in denial. If I had been, I would not have accepted her mild to moderate diagnosis, nor would I have accepted the referral to the Occupational Therapist. I would have just continued to hope for her to get well without taking any practical steps on my part.

One of the practical steps I took was booking a screening with an optometrist on Saturday to check her eyesight. I also booked a trial for her to start swimming, as per her OT's recommendation. Lastly, we were starting her OT lessons on Saturday. It felt like a lot of things, but they were necessary so she would not struggle later. It was better for us to address all these issues now rather than later.

So, this is me again asking you to seek help when you start suspecting anything concerning your child. It was better to be called names for being too much than to live with regrets.

Conversation with Occupational Therapist Katiso Ndumo

You are an occupational therapist; can you briefly share what occupational therapists do?

"According to the American Occupational Therapy Association, occupational therapists and occupational therapy assistants focus on the things people want and need to do in their daily lives. Occupational therapy intervention uses everyday life activities (occupations) to promote health, well-being, and the ability to participate in important activities. This includes any meaningful activity that a person wants to accomplish, such as taking care of themselves and their family, working, volunteering, and going to school, among many others (AOTA, 2012). I like to say we are all occupational beings, and OT allows us to engage in all the occupations, also known as activities of daily living, as optimally and independently as possible.

With children specifically, OTs help children with any delays in their developmental milestones, limitations such as learning difficulties, cognitive skills, decreased fine motor skills, physical strength, motor planning, etc."

What are some common misconceptions people have about occupational therapists?

- OT is for people with severe impairments, such as disabilities only.
- When someone is referred for OT, it means they are mentally unstable or incompetent.
- OT is mainly to help someone get a job or assist them with work-related tasks.
- OTs just keep patients busy.
- OT is the same as physiotherapy.
- OT is an easy profession.

You know that I struggled when my daughter was referred to an occupational therapist because I didn't think she needed one. Can you share some reasons why kids need occupational therapists?

- Children need occupational therapy because they are also occupational beings. The main activity or 'occupation' that children engage in is play.
- They have developmental milestones that need to be reached. Therefore, they need to be stimulated and encouraged to engage in appropriate activities that will allow them to develop well and thrive in these milestones. For example, before a child can sit at a desk and write, they

need to strengthen the fundamentals, such as postural tone, postural control, shoulder stability, forearm stability, core strength, and pelvic stability. This will enable the child to not tire easily when sitting at a desk and engaging in a task, allowing for better control in their activities.

- Children's sensory systems also need to be stimulated from infancy through toddler stage and into school-going age. This allows them to have regulated systems as they mature in age or when they start school, avoiding the constant urge to seek movement, also known as vestibular input.
- Children's brains keep developing and maturing, and at that tender age, it is crucial to build mentally, emotionally, physically, and psychologically fit individuals who will become a healthy generation for our ever-changing society.

How do we access an occupational therapist? Do we need a referral first, or can people contact you directly?

- In most cases, a referral from another healthcare professional, school setting, or work setting is ideal to know what challenges have been identified with the individual being referred.
- However, sometimes not all clients who consult with us have been seen elsewhere, so they come as self-referrals, which we also accept. Someone or a parent might identify a few things they or their child have challenges with and see it fit to see an OT.

What are some common signs that parents can look for to determine whether a child needs an occupational therapist?

- Children are different and develop in different ways, so while we don't compare children to each other, we look at how they are developing according to their developmental milestones. If a child is delayed in their milestones by six months or more, it is advisable to investigate consulting with an occupational therapist.
- When a child regresses in more than two milestones, such as stopping walking or stopping talking.
- When a child is very clumsy, always bumping into objects or dropping things.
- Difficulty following instructions and engaging in tasks.
- Difficulty concentrating or completing tasks.
- Hyperactivity, constantly seeking movement even when required to engage in a task.
- Sensory defensiveness to movement, not wanting to be moved, rocked, or go on slides and swings.
- Sensory defensiveness to tactile input, not wanting to touch certain textures or being irritated by name tags, clothing seams, and certain foods.
- A lack of enjoyment in play or being very passive, not wanting to engage in any play tasks.
- Limited fine motor skills, which involve the use of smaller muscles in the hands and fingers to manipulate objects or engage in tasks.

- Limited gross motor skills, which involve the use of larger muscles in the body to engage in tasks.
- Behavioural problems.
- Difficulty engaging in activities of daily living, such as feeding, bathing, dressing, and tying shoelaces, based on what is expected at that age.

As a parent going through OT with her child, how can I better support my child through the process?

- Encourage your child to be the best version of themselves. Explain to them that they are attending OT not because there is something wrong with them, but because we are all different and unique, and some children need extra support to improve their skills and reach their greatest potential.
- Please never compare your child to their peers; continue to love and embrace your child's abilities.
- Try not to overwhelm your child or put too much pressure on them because of the expectations you have in mind, but support them and help them through the journey by openly communicating with the therapists about what is working and not working for your child to better adjust their treatment intervention.
- Include the OT activities within the daily routines, as life can get very busy and hectic for working parents.

Any encouraging words for parents about to start this process or already going through it?

You are your child's greatest treasure; take care of yourself so that you can be better equipped to take care of them as they embark on this journey.

Woman Down

Today I went to the doctor for catching the flu, and I decided that I should attend to it before it became worse. While there, I shared with her how emotionally and physically tired I was. I had been doing well until she told me that I should not be hard on myself but should celebrate the fact that I realised I needed help for my child and continued to fight for her. When she said that, I couldn't help but cry. Perhaps you are going through the same, wondering if what you are doing is enough or focusing on your so-called mistakes. She encouraged me to buy a small cake to celebrate our progress so far, to celebrate all my efforts. That is my encouragement to you too; despite how we feel sometimes, the fact that we are still here fighting for our kids is worth celebrating. So, I urge you to go out and buy or bake yourself that muffin or cake and celebrate your progress so far. While there, I mentioned that I needed a referral to a professional to process everything with a neutral person. She gave me a card, which I planned to use. As much as I talked to different people, I felt that I would benefit from speaking to a professional. Lastly, my biggest takeaway from my consultation was that I should talk to my daughter about how we started our journey. If you remember, I shared how, before we discovered that she had a speech delay, I would get frustrated with her when it seemed that she was unable to say simple words. Even though we went through her physical healing, we never did the emotional one, and honestly, I never considered that she might be holding on to what happened. So, when she came back from school, that's what I did. I apologised for losing my temper with her, for not understanding that she had physical limitations that prevented her from understanding what I was saying. And you know what? She started crying, and I realised that she might have carried that pain and the incorrect belief that I blamed her for what was happening and that I was not proud of her. I thanked God that He brought that doctor to help me repair my relationship with my daughter and to help me heal her heart. You know what happened in the following days? Every day, she would randomly say, "Mama, I still forgive you." At first, I couldn't catch what she was forgiving me for, then she said, "For what you said," and I quickly replied, "Thank you for forgiving me." She smiled. I felt like every time she told me that she forgave me, it not only healed her but healed me too. Because the truth was that on this journey, despite our best intentions, we would sometimes lose our cool and say things that we did not mean. When those things happened, instead of beating myself up, I remembered to apologise to my child and then forgive myself. I was only human, and sometimes I would fail despite my best efforts.

New Session And Another Test

It was May 25th, and after attending her session, we quickly went to the optometrist. We were going to do a comprehensive eye screening, and if we were honest, besides the recommendation from a close family friend, what made me choose them was the fact that they accepted medical aid. That made a huge difference; whether they accepted medical aid or not was significant. My daughter was understandably nervous. I could only imagine how the constant tests made her feel, and I knew that this was nothing compared to other kids. As I said before, it didn't nullify our feelings. After doing the technical tests, she mentioned that there was nothing physically wrong with my daughter's eyesight that would hinder her from reading or writing. However, when we continued the tests, it seemed that she might need glasses to help her build her confidence when reading and writing. Though she wanted it to be a temporary solution until her eyesight was strengthened, I noticed how differently we reacted to her news. For her dad, it felt like progress because we knew what to attend to, while for me, it felt like a step backward—another thing to work on. I felt I was tired.

13

What If The Lord Revealed The Hidden Parts Of Your Child So That They Would Receive The Help That They Needed?

What if, instead of seeing another symptom unveiled as a bad thing, I saw it as an opportunity to attend to it? These were my thoughts last night as I put her to bed. As a Christian, I believed that the Lord knew my daughter before she was even formed in my womb. That meant the Lord saw her before she was created; He knew every part of her, even the ones that came as a surprise to me. So, instead of being afraid of what was next, I thought I could have faith to say, "Thank You, God, for revealing this to us." Don't get me wrong; I was not grateful for the diagnosis, but I was grateful that it was revealed to us so that we could attend to it. I was thankful that this was not hidden from us until she was older or became frustrated. I was grateful that we could provide her with the support she needed and give her the foundation necessary for a stronger finish. Reading Psalm 139:13-17 gave me the comfort I needed to face another day, to attend another speech therapy session, and to practise another OT exercise because God knew my daughter; nothing was and is hidden from Him. In His loving kindness, He was revealing it to us, and that day, I was grateful for that knowledge.

As I met with her teacher to provide feedback on her OT assessment and glasses, I was not feeling anxious about what was next but hopeful. The meeting went well, and I left feeling that I was not in denial. Yes, I needed a neutral person's confirmation because sometimes it was easy to doubt myself. Unlearning years of being told that women are emotional and illogical could do that to you. She shared that she had no concerns about my daughter's performance. I told her about the word-reversing, and she felt it was absolutely normal for her age. She believed my daughter was performing well in class, and all her challenges and wins were appropriate for her age. Based on her experience, she didn't think my daughter needed OT; however, she understood that they were specialists. Personally, for her, it seemed too soon and early for us to be concerned. She was happy with both my daughter's academic and social skills, though we would continue with OT and speech therapy. I was pleased that her teacher was fine with her progress at school. After the meeting, I took her to her speech session, where I met one of the moms who reached out online after I first shared our journey on social media. Through our interaction, she was able to take her child for a speech assessment, which led to discovering that her son's tongue was tied. After having the surgery, he was now doing speech therapy and doing well. Seeing her really touched my heart; it was a reminder that sharing your story makes a difference. There is someone who needed to know that they were not alone and that they were not crazy for feeling how they felt. That is why I am writing this book, hoping that as you read it, you would see your story in my story. I want you to feel less alone and more seen, to know that your story is valid and necessary, to trust your instincts again, and to listen to that still voice, even if it is scary doing that. As I had always said, one of the things I asked the Lord was that the pain and discomfort we went through as a family must at least help another child or adult; it must not be in vain. Seeing that mom reminded me that it was not in vain. Before anyone starts feeling the pressure to share their story, I want to clarify that this is not what I was advocating for. There is really no formula for how to manage this journey. Do what works for you and your family. If you don't want to share with others, that is totally okay, just as if you feel led to share with others. Both choices are okay. We have to be okay with our diversity.

Different Opinions

One thing about being on this journey is that you will hear different opinions, whether from your loved ones, strangers, or professionals. Sometimes the opinions will contradict each other, and you may not be sure which one is right or wrong. Instead of beating yourself up about which is true or false, I encourage you to give yourself the grace to change your mind. Allow yourself the grace to try new things; some will work out, while others may not be right for you. Occasionally, you will discover that new information is still being uncovered about your child's diagnosis. Sometimes, you will be among those who contribute to new research because of your experiences and the questions you ask. Other times, you may find that there is not enough information regarding your child's diagnosis. This had been my experience with mild to moderate speech delay; when I searched Google, I found limited information available, and I suppose that might be the reason why we did not uncover more. I mentioned to her therapist that when I heard "speech delay," I assumed her treatment plan would include hearing and speaking, so I did not expect it to involve occupational therapy. I also thought that once she had undergone the surgeries and attended speech therapy, she would be fine; however, that was not the case, hence the book. The therapist mentioned that most of the time, children with speech delays are often referred to an occupational therapist, and that with this diagnosis, some symptoms gradually emerge as the child grows and is exposed to different environments. Regarding the lack of information online, it is because, unlike other diagnoses, this is not considered severe, as in most cases, it usually resolves as the child undergoes various treatments before growing.

The End Of Term 2

We had come to the end of Term 2. Schools closed, and we received her report. She had done very well according to her report; what was sad was that I was unsure whether to rejoice or worry. There were a few areas she needed to work on, such as counting backwards from 20 to 0 and mastering our home address. I had not included the house number, so we needed to fix that. Her teacher had included alphabet flashcards to help all the children practise their letters in preparation for when they started to read. I was excited for her and all the new things she would experience; however, I was worried that she had too much work, and I could see that she felt a bit overwhelmed. Honestly, I also felt a bit overwhelmed with all the different exercises we had to do daily. Sometimes I forgot one of them and only realised as I was about to sleep that we hadn't done it. I thought she celebrated the fact that I sometimes forgot.

Our daily routine, excluding her normal activities, included her physical exercises in the morning before school. After school, it started with her physical exercise again, followed by arm exercises using therapy play dough. Then came her speech activities, her eye tracking (which most days I forgot, hence I decided to create an alarm for it), and lastly, her school homework. All of this had to be done between 4 pm and 6 pm before she started her bath, had dinner, and began her bedtime routine, finally going to sleep at 8 pm. At the end of the day, we really didn't have the energy or motivation to complete them. You might have been going through this yourself, where you didn't feel like doing another exercise, or perhaps your child was the one who didn't want to do another task. I completely understand; however, I believe that in this case, our feelings need to listen to our minds because we know that in the end, it will all be worth it. At least that is what I kept telling myself. One other thing that might have helped was asking for help if we had people who were willing to assist us. I taught them how to do the different exercises so that the burden didn't fall on me alone. I had noticed that she enjoyed it when we did the exercises together or when she took the lead as if she was teaching us. I incorporated this into our routine; she sometimes exercised with her brothers or her father, or I did it with her. To be honest, as much as the exercises were beneficial, the routine could become tiring and repetitive for a small child who wanted to have fun. I understood how she felt; however, as her mother, I needed to keep pushing, irrespective of how we felt, because sometimes the right things don't feel good in the moment.

Have you ever felt as though you were constantly correcting your children or overanalysing their actions?

That was how I felt most of the time. Unlike a mother whose child had never been diagnosed, I often took things more seriously. If she mispronounced a word, my immediate reaction was to wonder whether it was more serious than I thought. I felt the need to fix it immediately before it escalated. I was also aware that most children her age were not entirely fluent and still made mistakes, but because I now lived with the knowledge of her "mild to moderate speech delay," I unfortunately viewed most things through that lens. To be honest, it was exhausting—not only for me, but I was sure for her as well, as she couldn't just be herself without my corrections.

One thing that worried me was that the constant correcting might affect her confidence, and that was something I would hate. So, how could I find a balance? I was considering blocking off the weekends for fun, free from formal speech or occupational therapy exercises. We would still do those activities but in a way that she wouldn't be aware of it. It might look like having a dance party or engaging in "Mommy and Me" exercises, going to the park, or baking together while incorporating some of the skills we had learned. Ultimately, we don't want to raise children who don't enjoy their childhood. In our quest to help them reach their full potential, we need to ensure that we aren't inadvertently harming them in the process.

As schools closed, the school provided them with holiday work to complete at home, focusing on writing alphabets. This added another item to her already full schedule, so we had decided to stop doing the flashcards. We were now focusing on her school homework, occupational therapy exercises, and speech activities. For our current season, that would have to be more than enough.

14

🗨

Conversation with Speech Therapist Nazmeerah

"A speech therapist assesses and treats a variety of communicative disorders and challenges, including:

- Speech sound disorders
- Language delays or disorders
- Delayed communicative development
- Speech and language challenges due to a genetic condition, neurological condition, or disability
- Voice difficulties
- Literacy difficulties
- Auditory processing challenges

- Disturbances in speech and language following a stroke or head injury
- Stuttering
- Feeding difficulties

It can thus be seen that we work with individuals of all ages, from newborns to the elderly."

Do we need a referral to see a speech therapist?

"You do not need a referral. We are often the first point of contact for parents who are concerned about their child's speech and language development. We generally guide parents with further recommendations, such as whether a child may need to see an occupational therapist for gross/fine motor or perceptual concerns, or if a neurodevelopmental specialist should evaluate them for pervasive developmental disorders, such as autism. We also advise parents on pursuing optometry and audiology evaluations.

Sometimes, as a society, we might feel like more children are being diagnosed. What do you think is the reason for that?

Parents today have much greater access to information at the click of a button. Social media has raised awareness about apparent difficulties and the various interventions available. Additionally, professionals have begun adopting a more holistic approach, engaging in rich and diverse referrals to enhance a child's overall development. Furthermore, an increasing number of children are presenting with challenges due to the lifestyle that millennial and Gen-Z parents have adopted. Excessive screen time and limited social/playtime are on the rise, contributing to a significant increase in developmental delays.

In the context of our current world, what should parents look for to determine whether to seek help?

"If you are even slightly concerned, DO AN ASSESSMENT! Early intervention is critical in ensuring better developmental and communicative outcomes for children. The following milestones are important indicators of communication; any deviations in this regard may warrant a speech and language assessment:

- Saying a few true words between 12 and 15 months
- Combining words to form short phrases by 18 months
- Having a steadily growing vocabulary
- Developing emerging social and pragmatic skills
- Achieving steady reading and spelling skills from Grade R to 1
- Understanding social cues
- Exhibiting fluent and smooth speech
- Following instructions of increasing complexity
- Expressing needs using complete sentences"

> Any encouragement for parents whose children are attending sessions?

"Firstly, well done to you as a parent for taking a step in the right direction. You are doing the best you can, and you should be very proud of yourself. The journey may seem long, and the road may be challenging, but you will witness progress and change. Remain consistent, persevere, and put in the effort as a family regarding carryover activities. A strong support system is vital for your child; they pick up on your emotions, energy, and investment. Take care of yourself so that you can care for them. Remember, we are therapists, but many of us are also mothers. We understand the journey all too well, and we are here to support and guide you through it all."

God Made Me This Way

We were busy doing her exercises, and for some reason, she really doesn't enjoy the playdough activities. I think it's because her dough is the therapy kind, which is a bit hard and requires her to use strength, unlike the regular playdough that most kids love. She randomly said to me, "Mama, my fingers are flexible." I innocently replied, "Yes, they are." She then remarked, "Yours are not," and I agreed with her. Following that, she said, "Mama, God made my fingers flexible, so God made me this way. I do not need to fix my fingers."

One thing about my daughter is that she often expresses unexpected thoughts. Honestly, I did not know how to respond, so I did what most moms would do: I laughed and mumbled something about her needing to do her exercises to help her. You might wonder how she knows her fingers are flexible; it came from her first feedback with her OT. To illustrate what she meant about her bones, she used her fingers to show me and explained that they are more flexible than ours. I guess she is still holding onto the idea that she is doing her exercises to fix her flexible fingers, but as she said, there is nothing wrong with her fingers because God made her like that.

I talked to a friend about being mindful that while doing all these interventions to help her, I don't end up harming her self-confidence. I want my daughter to know that she is loved and appreciated just as she is. I love her flexible fingers; I love all of her just as she is right now. Everything we are doing is to make life easier for her as she grows; we want her to show up confidently in this world. However, I never want her to feel that we are doing all of this to "fix" her or that there is something wrong with her because even if she did not do all these things, she is still our blessing, the daughter we prayed for. One of the affirmations we use is, "My family loves me, and I am enough."

So, this is my encouragement: as you navigate this journey, do not forget to affirm your child. The truth is that sometimes it is easier to focus on what needs to be worked on and overlook the miracle that they are. We celebrate the fact that they are alive, and despite the odds being against them, they continue to fight and find new ways of being, which is remarkable. The fact that they are still here despite their diagnosis or that they have discovered other ways of communicating and living beyond the "normal" channels is worth celebrating.

I did a live recording on Instagram with Tasmin, and one of the points she mentioned was the issue of "neuroplasticity," explaining how the brain is able to create new pathways for doing things, and I have seen this in action. Before her surgery, she used non-verbal cues to convey her messages. I am sure you also have your own examples of how your child does things differently from what you were used to, but somehow, they are able to achieve their goals.

Sometimes Healing is Gradual

As we approach my daughter's sixth birthday, I can't help but reflect on our journey so far. I am grateful for the little girl who has changed my life for the better. Yesterday, on the 20th, we attended her OT session, and afterwards, her therapist shared how well she is doing. She is physically and emotionally strong, and her writing and identification of letters have also improved. I left the session feeling encouraged and excited for her.

After that, we went to an open day at her school, where she was part of the group that performed a musical item for the new parents. Seeing her confidently perform with other kids and play with them afterward warms my heart. These are the things I prayed for—to see her interact with others, find her own way, and build relationships. I wanted to witness her playing with other children and advocating for herself without worrying whether they could hear or understand her.

On our way home in an Uber, she had a conversation with the driver, and I must say, my Mommy's heart was so proud. When we started this journey, my prayer for her was that she would be able to navigate life independently. We are not 100% there yet, but there is so much progress.

This is the thing I keep noticing on this journey: it is essential to pause and reflect on the process. It is all too easy to focus solely on the challenges and forget to acknowledge and celebrate the triumphs. My baby can say so many words that she didn't know last year, and that is worth celebrating. She can hold conversations with us and strangers, and she is doing well at school. Just this weekend, we rehearsed a poem—something I would have never thought she could do. She can memorise things and remember them.

As I type this, a small voice reminds me that she sometimes mixes up the word order in her sentences. This highlights the challenge of remembering that two things can be true and worth celebrating. I can celebrate the progress while continuing to work on areas that need attention. So today, I choose to celebrate the progress. I celebrate her strength and resilience. I celebrate the blessing that is my daughter, the girl who has reminded me of my inner strength and resilience.

CHAPTER FOURTEEN

She has taught me to trust my voice again and to share my opinions without fear of what others might say or think. I hope you are also learning to trust yourself as you continue on this journey. Celebrate the mother you are and the one you are becoming each day. Celebrate how you have fought for your child and continue to advocate for them. I celebrate you, and I am proud of the woman you are.

15

For the One Who No Longer Trusts Her Intuition

How to Trust Yourself Again as a Mother

To further explore this topic, I reached out to other mothers about their parenting journey. I asked each of them the same questions, allowing them to share their stories and insights.

Here are the questions to also help you reflect on your parenting journey:

> Have you ever doubted your intuition or gut feeling when it comes to raising your children?

Many mothers find themselves second-guessing their instincts, especially in a world filled with unsolicited advice and differing parenting philosophies.

This doubt can stem from various sources, such as negative experiences, criticism from others, or overwhelming information on parenting trends. It's important to remember that intuition is a natural part of being a parent, shaped by your unique experiences and knowledge of your child.

What do you think led to that doubt?

Reflect on the circumstances that may have contributed to your loss of confidence. Perhaps it was a challenging situation where you felt unsupported, or maybe it was a moment when you questioned your decisions after hearing conflicting opinions from family, friends, or online sources. Recognising these influences is the first step in reclaiming your trust in yourself.

What helped you rediscover your faith in your intuition?

Rebuilding trust in your instincts often requires a conscious effort. Start by reflecting on past experiences where your intuition guided you successfully. Consider keeping a journal to document moments when you trusted your gut and the positive outcomes that followed. Engaging in self-care practices, seeking support from other mothers, and surrounding yourself with positive influences can also help. Remember that every parent makes mistakes; these moments are learning opportunities rather than failures.

Trusting your intuition as a mother is a journey that may have ups and downs, but it is essential for your growth and the well-being of your children. Embrace your unique voice and experiences, and allow yourself to celebrate the moments when you listen to your instincts.

I hope the following stories encourage you and help reignite the belief in your instincts as a mother

Nomsa Mzozo
Mom of Three | Digital Content Creator

My gut feeling has not failed me yet as a mother. It's the one thing I trust, especially in my journey through motherhood. Whenever I've sensed something amiss, I've often been correct. Even when I'm unsure, I don't dismiss that initial feeling of intuition as false. Instead, I view it as a warning, prompting me to be vigilant about potential "dangers" that may arise. This instinct has guided me through numerous challenges, reminding me that my intuition is a valuable ally in parenting.

I have come to understand that a mother's intuition is a powerful tool, reinforced by my experiences with my own mother and grandmother. Whenever their intuition alerted them to something concerning me, it was almost always accurate. Even if I initially doubted some situations, deep down, I knew they were right. This legacy of intuition has inspired me to trust my own instincts as a mother, instilling confidence in my ability to care for and protect my children.

Bathabile Magethi

Mom of Four | Speaker | Founder of Visionary Women

Have you ever doubted your intuition or gut feeling when it comes to raising your kids?

"Doubt often feels like an inevitable part of motherhood. From the early days of worrying about whether I've fed them enough milk to second-guessing myself for excluding them from certain experiences, it can be overwhelming. However, what has truly transformed my approach is consistently asking the Holy Spirit to guide my steps. After all, the Word of God reminds us that a double-minded man will not receive anything from Him (James 1:7-8). Now, I allow the peace from the Holy Spirit to guide my decisions, striving to stay in tune with Him as I navigate the challenges of parenting."

What do you think led to that?

"My initial doubts stemmed from not fully trusting God to lead me in parenting my children. He is their true Parent and Creator (Genesis 1:28), while I am merely a steward on His behalf. I've come to realise that He desires even greater things for them than I could ever imagine. This understanding has helped me shift my

136

perspective and rely on His wisdom rather than my own insecurities."

What helped you rediscover faith in your intuition again?

"I would describe this journey as cultivating an intimate relationship with Christ. Through the Holy Spirit, I have access to the truth about what I need to do. The closer I draw to Christ, the clearer my understanding becomes, and the more direction I receive. Keeping in step with the Holy Spirit has been a game changer for all matters concerning our children, families, and life in general (Galatians 5:25)."

Logracia Ekstein
Digital Creator | Mom of One

> Have you ever doubted your intuition or gut feeling when it comes to raising your kids?

"Yes, I have. I often found myself second-guessing my choices, especially when they diverged from what I saw or heard other mothers doing. For example, when my son was younger and prescribed medication for an illness, I followed the doctor's orders and administered all his medicine at once. However, I overheard a few mothers saying they preferred to wait at least 15 minutes before giving a different type of medication. This led me to question whether I was overwhelming his system with too much medication. Concerned, I consulted our doctor, who reassured me that my approach was perfectly fine. Despite this confirmation, I still struggled with self-doubt.

Another instance where I questioned my decisions was when I encouraged my son to complete his homework independently. Once he was able to comprehend the instructions, I stopped sitting with him while he worked. Instead, I encouraged him to ask for help when needed. While I would still check his homework afterward, I felt uneasy about not actively helping him. At that time, this approach was not common, and I frequently doubted whether I was making the right choice."

What do you think led to that?

"In both cases, my doubts stemmed from listening to others and comparing their approaches to mine. I was raising our son differently than how I had been raised, and without a clear blueprint or prior experience to guide me, I often lacked confidence in my decisions. The pressure to conform to the norms I observed around me only amplified my uncertainty."

What helped you rediscover faith in your intuition again?

Over time, I learned to accept that I am a different kind of mother with my own beliefs and values, which may not always align with those of others. This understanding allowed me to embrace my unique parenting style. I also started praying for guidance on how to be a better mother, which significantly improved my confidence. Additionally, I sought therapy to address my personal struggles, ensuring that I do not transfer my fears onto my son. Recognising that I am doing my best has been incredibly liberating and has helped me trust my instincts more fully.

Tabea Mngadi
Personal Development Coach | Mom of Two

> Have you ever doubted your intuition or gut feeling when it comes to raising your kids?

"Yes, I have. Reflecting on my parenting journey, particularly the season when I was a single parent before marrying and forming a family in alignment with God's design, brings to mind one significant moment. As a young single parent who had endured a challenging previous relationship, I faced a pivotal decision when my then-partner entered my life. We both realised that our relationship was serious, which meant I needed to consider introducing my son to him. This was a moment that caused me to wrestle with my intuition. I had to decide whether to lift the boundary I had maintained for so long and take the risk of allowing my partner to get to know my son, despite not having any guarantees about what the future might hold."

What do you think led to that?

"Upon reflection, the primary force behind my questioning of my intuition was fear. I grappled with the fear of the unknown, the concern that my son and my partner might not bond, and the haunting worry of "What if we break up? What will happen if a strong bond develops between them?" Additionally, I was carrying the weight of past trauma inflicted by a male figure who had failed to model what a good man should be. The thought of giving another man a chance at building a relationship with my son, and relinquishing control over that situation, was daunting at first."

What helped you rediscover faith in your intuition again?

"What ultimately helped me regain trust in my intuition was the knowledge that my partner was deeply rooted in Christ and had a genuine fear of the Lord. I had prayed for him long before we met, writing a heartfelt letter to God detailing the qualities I desired in a man, including the ability to be a father figure to my child. I had to remind myself that embracing love again and allowing God to restore my life meant I needed to walk by faith and not by sight.

Taking the risk to open those boundaries was essential for me to determine if my partner was truly the man I believed he was. If God intended for restoration in my life, part of that process involved demonstrating, through practical experience, whether my partner could be a good father to my son. I recognised that this could not happen if I kept them apart any longer. Building a rapport between them was a crucial part of the courtship process, allowing them the time to connect organically. This understanding was vital as I considered the implications of marriage and what it would mean for our family dynamic.

In the end, I had to release myself from the spirit of fear and trust in God's will for my life, which included creating a healthy and functional family."

Boledi Makatlaneng

Psychology Graduate | Mental Health Advocate | Mom of Three

Have you ever doubted your intuition or gut feeling when it comes to raising your kids?

"In the few instances where I have doubted my instinct as a mother, life has quickly reminded me not to compromise what my gut tells me. Even when my intuition didn't seem to make sense at the time, it consistently proved to be correct. This experience taught me to trust my instincts early in my parenting journey."

What do you think led to that?

"One major incident stands out when I ignored my gut feeling, despite knowing deep down that I was making the wrong decision. As a new mom, I found myself surrounded by women who had been mothers for much longer than I had. In that moment, I chose to avoid conflict and didn't want to come across as a "know-it-all" to those I sought help and guidance from. However, I knew very well that I wasn't making the right choice and was, in fact, betraying my instincts."

What helped you rediscover faith in your intuition again?

The consequences of not following my gut in that situation led me to make a promise to myself: I would never dishonour my instincts like that again. To support my journey in learning to trust my voice, I implemented several tools:

- **Self-Discovery**: I dedicated time to getting to know myself better. Investing in personal development, reading insightful books, and establishing clear boundaries all contributed to my growth.

- **Mindfulness Practices**: Engaging in activities such as meditation, regular exercise, therapy, and spiritual practices like fasting helped me centre myself. These practices not only grew my confidence but also strengthened my ability to trust my gut when I felt grounded and centred.

By nurturing my self-awareness and creating a strong foundation through various practices, I've learned to listen to my intuition as a guiding force in my parenting journey.

Leanne Dlamini

Founder of EndGirlHate & Life Designed By Her | Mom of Two

Have you ever doubted your intuition or gut feeling when it comes to raising your kids?

"Absolutely. Motherhood and parenting do not come with a handbook or a set of instructions to help us navigate this journey. From the moment I had my first child to the arrival of my second, I found myself doubting my intuition and second-guessing my decisions constantly. I often wondered: Am I making the right choice? Is what I'm feeling just a fleeting emotion? I tend to be an overthinker, and this tendency amplifies during my parenting journey. I find myself making things seem bigger than they are at times, always having to talk myself down from the ledge and reframing worst-case scenarios that lead me to doubt myself and my instincts."

What do you think led to your self-doubt?

"As I mentioned, there's no parenting handbook, and every parent is essentially learning through trial and error. Each child is different, so the experience varies every time. This constant worry creeps in, especially when I recall how things went with my first child. In different stages of parenthood, new doubts arise. With newborns, there are unique challenges, then you transition to dealing with toddlers, tweens, teens, and eventually young adults. Each new phase leads me to question whether I am doing the right thing, especially since we've never been in that situation before. This lack of guidance can often lead to self-doubt."

What helped you rediscover faith in your intuition regarding parenting?

"I came to the realization that God equipped me for this parenting journey. I was always meant to be their mother, which reassures me and boosts my confidence. Knowing that God trusts me with these children allows me to embrace my role, regardless of whether I feel I'm making the right decisions. Children do not need a perfect parent; they just need a mother who shows up as she was created to be.

I strive to raise my children with love, consistency, support, and understanding, remaining a stable presence in their lives and their biggest cheerleader every day. Mistakes are part of the process—we all make them—but remembering that God has equipped me for this journey gives me peace. Each parent's journey is unique, and while some may hide their struggles better than others, we all face challenges. Knowing that I have the tools to raise my children reassures me. Ultimately, I focus on trying my best, being the best version of myself, and maintaining my connection to God. Staying grounded in prayer as I raise Zani-Lee and Zaya Rose has been pivotal in centring me as a mother."

Refilwe Ndhlovu
Author | Mom of One

> **Have you ever doubted your intuition or gut feeling when it comes to raising your kids? What do you think led to that?**

"Yes, I have definitely experienced self-doubt, and sometimes I still do. This is particularly true when there is a lot of "noise" around me—when life feels overwhelming, and I am struggling to meet various demands. During these challenging seasons, the natural flow of life gets disrupted, tipping the balance and leaving me feeling unsettled."

> **What helped you rediscover faith in your intuition again?**

"I found that leaning in has been transformative. There is immense power in connecting with what uplifts me. For me, that is my faith in God and the understanding that, as a parent, I am merely a vessel and earthly guide. God is the orchestrator of my daughter's life, and leaning into Him has been crucial in helping me regain trust in my intuition.

I've also learned to acknowledge my feelings. Like anyone else, when I'm not at my best, my results suffer. I've recognised the importance of allowing myself the space to be still without the shame of judgement. This practice of self-acknowledgement has enabled me to embrace the transformational power of vulnerability in parenting, allowing me to have open conversations with my daughter about my fears, concerns, and ideas while soliciting her feedback.

Additionally, I've made it a point to be intentional about grounding activities, such as spending time in nature, being playful with my daughter, taking naps, or walking barefoot. These investments in self-care are always worthwhile. When my mind is clear, my discernment sharpens, and I no longer feel confused about my actions or the lessons I need to impart in raising my daughter."

Katlego Moagi
Digital Creator | Mom of Two

Have you ever doubted your intuition or gut feeling when it comes to raising your kids?

"Absolutely, I have. Motherhood is a journey filled with uncertainty, and there have been numerous occasions where I've found myself questioning my instincts. It's an ongoing struggle, especially in a world that often presents a façade of calm and control. When I sense something is off—whether it's my child's behaviour or a situation that feels uncomfortable—I sometimes hesitate to act on those feelings."

What led to that doubt?

"A significant factor in my doubt is the pressure to conform to societal norms and expectations. In moments of concern, I often find myself surrounded by other parents who seem entirely at ease, which can amplify my self-doubt. For example, if I notice something concerning about my child and everyone else appears relaxed, I begin to question whether I'm overreacting. I worry that I might be perceived as dramatic or paranoid, leading me to dismiss my instincts in favour of what seems to be a collective calm. This internal conflict creates a cycle of second-guessing and anxiety."

What emotions did you experience when you ignored your intuition?

"When I ignore my intuition, I often experience a profound sense of guilt. It's a nagging feeling that lingers in the back of my mind, reminding me that I had an instinct to act differently. This guilt intensifies when I reflect on how I could have potentially prevented an issue by listening to my gut feeling. The knowledge that I might have sidestepped a problem adds weight to my emotions. Each time I dismiss my intuition, it not only erodes my confidence as a mother but also deepens my resolve to trust my instincts in the future. The desire to avoid guilt and regret becomes a powerful motivator for me to pay closer attention to my feelings moving forward.

Ultimately, these experiences have taught me the importance of listening to my intuition. They have reinforced the belief that my instincts are valid and deserve to be acknowledged. I'm learning to trust myself more, knowing that I am my child's best advocate and that my feelings hold significance in our parenting journey."

Tiyiselani Ndhlovu
Digital Creator | Mom of Four

Have you ever doubted your intuition or gut feeling when it comes to raising your kids?

Sadly, yes, I have experienced moments of doubt in my parenting journey. Parenting is an incredibly personal and often challenging path, and there have been times when I questioned my instincts, especially when faced with difficult situations involving my children.

What led to that doubt?

A significant factor contributing to my doubt has been external influences and criticism from others. My parenting approach has always differed from the way I was raised, which naturally brought its share of scrutiny. While I have always been committed to standing my ground and following my beliefs, I found that when I started encountering challenges with my kids, the weight of that criticism became harder to bear. It created a ripple effect in my confidence as a mother. Instead of trusting my instincts, I began to second-guess my decisions, worrying that maybe I wasn't doing things right. This struggle led me to question whether my parenting style was adequate or effective, particularly when faced with resistance or setbacks.

What helped you regain faith in your intuition?

Over time, I've learned that age and maturity play crucial roles in building confidence in my parenting decisions. With each passing year and as I navigated various challenges, I began to see the positive outcomes of the choices I made for my children. Witnessing the fruits of my efforts, such as my children developing into compassionate, confident individuals, has reassured me that my intuition and instincts are valid. The journey has taught me that while outside opinions can be loud, it's essential to tune into my own voice and trust the decisions I make for my family. Each success, no matter how small, reinforces my belief that I am capable and that my unique approach to parenting is indeed valuable.

In embracing this journey of self-discovery and learning, I've grown more resolute in my parenting philosophy. While I may face challenges and criticism, I now understand that my intuition is a vital guide in raising my children. As a mother, I am learning to trust that I know what's best for my family, which ultimately empowers me to continue striving for growth and connection with my children.

The Journey Continues

My prayer is that as you read this book, it will help you reconnect with the little girl who was confident, fearless, and trusted her inner knowing. I hope you will forgive yourself for the times you did not listen to her or for not trusting her instincts. I pray that you will also forgive her for not knowing better or for knowing better but not applying those lessons.

As you read, may you find yourself reconnecting with that part of yourself again. Remember, you are the best parent for your child, and the Lord knew that they needed you to navigate this life. I hope you take note of your progress and celebrate the fact that you are no longer where you used to be. While you may not have reached your ultimate goal yet, the simple fact that you are moving forward is worth celebrating.

If you have recently received a diagnosis, I hope this book helps you feel less alone and reminds you that help is available. May it serve not only as a resource for yourself but also for your family. Remember, you are the expert on your child, and may you never doubt your knowledge, even when it feels like what you know does not make sense.

I hope that one day my daughter will share her story from her own perspective. Until then, see you on social media and offline. Please pray for us as we pray for you.

Embracing Uncertainty with Faith

As we conclude this chapter of our journey together, we acknowledge the uncertainties that lie ahead. The path of parenting, especially when faced with challenges, can often feel daunting and filled with questions. Yet, amid this uncertainty, we hold steadfast to our faith—faith in ourselves, in our children, and in the unwavering love that binds us as parents.

Trusting our instincts as mothers is paramount. We must not leave the fate of our children in the hands of society's opinions or what it tries to impose on us. The new breed of parenting requires boldness—the courage to fight for our children unapologetically. It's about embracing our unique parenting styles, making choices that align with our values, and being brave enough to acknowledge that mistakes will happen. Ultimately, we will never regret following our gut instincts, for they guide us toward what is best for our children.

Our hope for our children is a bright light guiding us through the darkest days. Each child is a unique gift, full of potential and promise. As we nurture and support them, we foster resilience and strength that will empower them to face their own challenges. Together, we dream of a future where our children can thrive, embracing their individuality and achieving their dreams.

In this journey, it is important to remember that we are not alone. The power of community is profound. By coming together as parents, we can create support groups where we can share our experiences, fears, and triumphs. These connections remind us that we are part of a larger tapestry of love and understanding.

Together, we can provide encouragement, share resources, and lift each other up during tough times, reinforcing the notion that we are stronger when we unite.

While navigating medical bills can be a source of frustration, we also recognize the invaluable gifts that specialists bring to our lives. Their expertise provides hope and guidance, illuminating the path forward. They help us understand our children's needs better and equip us with tools to support their growth and development.

We must also honour the role of supportive families, including siblings, parents, and those who are walking this journey alone. Their love and involvement can make all the difference. A sibling's encouraging words, a grandparent's wisdom, or a friend's listening ear can provide comfort and strength. For parents navigating this journey solo, know that you are not alone. Your efforts and resilience are commendable, and you are deserving of support and compassion.

As we step into the future, let us carry these sentiments with us: faith amid uncertainty, hope for our children, the strength of community, the value of expertise, and the power of family support. Together, we will continue to navigate this journey, uplifting one another and embracing the beautiful chaos of parenthood.

Recap – The Experts

For quick reference, revisit the valuable insights shared by our experts throughout the book. Paediatrician, Occupational Therapist, Speech Therapist, and Social Worker.

See below pages for the conversations.

Dr Natasha Zechner – Paediatrician.....................................71

Conversation with Social Worker – Disabilities: Bulelwa
Mahura..90

Conversation with Occupational Therapist Katiso Ndumo......108

Conversation with Speech Therapist Nazmeerah...................124